The Freedom Diet

JESSICA BLACK, N.D.

The Freedom Diet

Lower Blood Sugar,

Lose Weight,

& Change Your Life

in 60 Days

TURNER
PUBLISHING COMPANY

Turner Publishing Company
424 Church Street • Suite 2240 • Nashville, Tennessee 37219
445 Park Avenue • 9th Floor • New York, New York 10022
www.turnerpublishing.com

The Freedom Diet: Lower Blood Sugar, Lose Weight, and Change Your Life in 60 Days

Cover design: Patrick Cabral and Maddie Cothren
Book design: Glen Edelstein

Library of Congress Cataloging-in-Publication Data
Black, Jessica.
The freedom diet : lower blood sugar, lose weight and change your life in 60 days / by Dr. Jessica Black.
    pages cm
  ISBN 978-1-68162-117-3 (pbk.)
1. Diet therapy--Popular works. 2. Nutrition--Popular works. 3. Self-care, Health--Popular works.
4. Food preferences. 5. Weight loss--Popular works. I. Title.
  RA784.B5513 2016
  613.2--dc23
                                    2015030299
Printed in the United States of America
10 9 8 7 6 5 4 3 2 1

Contents

Preface   *ix*

Acknowledgements   *xiii*

PART 1: *What Is Affecting Health Today?*   *1*

CHAPTER 1: *The True Definition of Health*   *3*

The Importance of Diet   5

The Problems with Our Current Lifestyle Habits   9

More Media Means New Issues   17

Lack of Sleep   20

Dietary Imbalances   21

Our Environment Is No Longer Clean   39

Quality of Grown Food   41

We Can't Meet All Our Needs with Supplements   43

The Importance of Children's Health on Their Future   45

CHAPTER 2: *Gastrointestinal Health Is Essential to Survival*   *49*

Probiotics in the Gastrointestinal Tract   50

The GI Tract Is Our First Immune System   51

The GI Tract's Role in Emotional Health   51

CHAPTER 3: *Inflammation's Impact on Health*   *53*

Predominant Illnesses in Our Society and throughout the World   53

Inflammation's Influence on Illness and Health 58
Inflammation at the Cellular Level 59
Inflammation and Chronic Diseases 66
The Harm in Chronic Use of Anti-Inflammatory
    Medications 67

CHAPTER 4: *The Importance of Blood Sugar* 69
Insulin Resistance and Metabolic Syndrome 69
Glucose Problems in Nondiabetics 72
Diabetes 74
Diabetic Medications 82

CHAPTER 5: *Blood Sugar and Its Relation
to Inflammation* 91
Current Diet Leads to Elevated Blood Sugar and Health
    Issues 91
Cooking Foods All Wrong 93

CHAPTER 6: *Obesity* 97
The Causes of Obesity 97

CHAPTER 7: *The Hormone Symphony* 101
Hypothalamus, the Director 102
Pituitary, the Mother 103
Thyroid, the Protector 104
Adrenal Glands, the Adaptors 112
Gonads, the Sex Glands 113
Pineal Gland, the Balancer 120
Vitamin D, the Immune Modulator 121

CHAPTER 8: *Other Health Risks: Are You at Risk for
Chronic Inflammation, Heart Disease, Cancer,
or Diabetes?* 123
Important Testing to Evaluate Your Risks 124

Red Flags 134

Statin Drugs—Should We Use Them? 136

Diabetes and Lipids and Increased Risk for Alzheimer's
Disease 137

Current Lifestyle and Dietary Habits Age Us and Lead to
Chronic Illness 139

PART 2: *The Freedom Diet* 141

CHAPTER 9: *Changing Your Diet for Better Health* 143

Paradigms of Medicine 143

You Really Are What You Eat 149

Foods to Include 153

Foods to Avoid 155

CHAPTER 10: *Habits to Include* 159

Sleep 160

Exercise 162

Mediation or Stress Relief 165

Nutrition for the Mind 166

Water Intake 171

Dietary Hygiene 173

CHAPTER 11: *Habits to Avoid* 177

Watching Television 177

Negative Thinking 178

Spending Time with Unhealthy People 178

Toxic Exposure 179

Self-Medicating with Substances 185

Overeating 186

Chart of Habits to Avoid and Include 189

CHAPTER 12: *The Supplement Program* 191

Breakfast or Lunch Supplements   191
Between Meals   191
Lunch or Dinner Supplements   191

CHAPTER 13: *Getting Prepared in the Kitchen*   193
Be Prepared and Don't Be Afraid   193
Navigating Food Choices   194
Food Items to Keep on Hand/Shopping List   197
Making Healthy Eating Easier   198
Measurement Conversions   201

CHAPTER 14: *Sample Freedom Diet Recipes*   203
Breakfast   305
Lunch   211
Dinner   219
Beverages   227
Snacks   232

CHAPTER 15: *Beyond 30 Days*   235
Foods to Try   235

CHAPTER 16: *Troubleshooting the Diet*   237
Medication Changes   237
Blood Sugar Still Too High   238
Blood Sugar Dipping Too Low   240
Not Eating Enough   240
Cravings   241
Eating Out   242

Afterword   245
Endnotes   247
Recommended Websites and Books   255
Index   263

Preface

The food revolution is here and can be confusing to navigate. With dietary suggestions coming from all directions, one must be able to search through all these suggestions and come up with the plan that is the best fit. Not all the recent fad diets are the same, but they have the same thing in common: their suggestions are trying to make you healthier. The fact is, if you pay attention to what is going into your body, then many of these food suggestions can be valid. No matter what diet you choose, the most important part is getting rid of the "fluff," the foods that carry with them a lot of calories without nutritional benefit. My advice to you is to search until you find what works best for you.

I love food. I love cooking and tasting and preparing creations in the kitchen. So when someone says to me I can't have something, my initial reaction is "WHAT?"

I don't want to have to restrict anything from my delicious goodness of a recipe. But if I must change things in my diet to help improve my health, then I guess I will. I have found that after practicing and seeing thousands of patients, I know what is out there for health issues, and I want to prevent myself and my patients from going down the same path of poor dietary and lifestyle choices that promote chronic diseases such as heart disease and various other ailments.

The Freedom Diet started in my office years ago when I was trying to figure out the fastest way to get a patient's blood sugar down. I had a patient who was a bus driver for the school system. She loved her job and she loved the children whom she drove daily. She came in after her blood sugar registered an alarming number. Her superiors discussed the health issue with her and let her know that if her blood sugar did not get under control within 30 days, she would be terminated. This was rather harsh and a rather short time frame to work within. We went to work and I came up with this diet and a supplement plan for her. She was an amazing subject to try the diet on because of her motivation to stay with the children. Her blood sugar levels came down significantly in a 30-day period, and she was still able to ride with her children.

When we first began the diet, we called it something like "blood sugar regulation diet." It was boring. One day, one of my patients was commenting on the diet and kiddingly called it "Freedom." She explained that even though the diet felt restrictive, it gave her freedom to do things she couldn't do previously in her unhealthy state. The name stuck, and to this day, we call it the Freedom Diet. Not because dieters can eat what they want, but because they become "free" to experience an unlimited amount of joy and improved health after being on the diet for a few months. They curb their sugar addictions, their mood improves, energy improves, sleep improves, pain improves, they lose weight, and they improve their blood sugar and lipid levels. Because of this, the diet has a truly "anti-aging" aspect to it, which will be discussed in depth later on in the book.

I have been using this rather strict diet for a long time with my patients to help improve blood sugars. When they adhere to this diet, along with making lifestyle changes and adding supplements, we can see fasting blood sugars drop dramatically in most patients. Everyone who adopts this diet sees a positive change. Most people will have more energy, better moods, and a better response to regular medical therapies. For years I have prescribed the anti-inflammatory diet to patients, but I realized that for a certain subset of patients, particularly those with diabetes, something stricter was needed at first to initiate a larger change in the body. This diet was originally only prescribed to diabetics to lower blood sugar, but over time it has transformed into a diet for wellness. It is a pure, "slow down the aging process," incredible diet that makes people feel well and begins to stimulate the regenerative processes within the body. To achieve significant changes in wellness, sometimes we need to take bigger leaps in our willingness to change. I won't lie, this diet is difficult, but it does have an end in sight, and then we can convert the diet into an easier to follow plan for the future. All I am asking for is 60 days of dedicated commitment so that you are able to begin changing the patterns that created ill health in the first place.

In a world of significant toxicities, sedentary habits, and poor dietary choices, the 60 days to freedom is a commitment you will never regret. Not only will this plan help you improve your health during the 60 days, it will help you convert some of your most unhealthy habits into healthier ones. Break your addictions, change your thinking, and eat healthy without counting calories for the rest of your life.

The more that I have studied sugar and its effect on the body, the more I have come to feel extremely strongly about this program. Not only does sugar impact future diabetes and cardiovascular health, it also largely impacts the rate at which we age. Increased amounts of blood sugars over long periods of time create an excess of oxidative stress in the body. Oxidative stress causes damage to arteries and many important tissues in the body and is directly related to aging. Sugar directly increases how much oxidative load your body encounters. The more oxidative damage that occurs within the body, the faster the aging process occurs. We will discuss further throughout the book oxidative damage, what it is, and what causes it, in addition to types of sugars and how we are consuming them in our diets.

I have put thousands of patients on this particular diet and program and have seen profound results when followed diligently and correctly. This 60-day program can be particularly helpful in reducing aging, diabetes, chronic infections of any type, arthritis, allergies, gastrointestinal issues, and more.

Acknowledgments

The special people whom I encounter day-to-day touch my life in unique ways. I am very thankful to my patients for teaching me so much about health and life struggles, and for having the confidence in me to willingly adopt my suggestions and prescriptions for health.

I thank all my staff and patients for their understanding and patience when my schedule was sometimes booked for months because of the time I spent growing as a writer and working to develop this program. I appreciate my patients' willingness to have doctor visits with my resident physicians as I worked to share this important program with the world.

I am thankful to my operations manager, Carrie Berreth, for her hard work and dedication to making sure our clinics run smoothly while I spend less time in them. I am so thankful to my business partner and husband, Jason, who has willingly increased his schedule to help as many people as possible improve their wellness.

I cannot say enough about my resident physicians, who have worked hard and taken up the additional patient load to allow me to spend time writing and preparing this book. Thank you to Dr. Colleen Tyler and Dr. Heather Crabtree for being competent, compassionate physicians and for using this time to grow as individuals as well as doctors.

Also, thank you to all the patients who have adhered faithfully to the Freedom Diet for 60 days or more! Thank you for showing me that this plan in fact does work at lowering blood sugars, improving health, and giving patients a true sense of well-being.

And special thanks to our loving nanny, Elisa Emley, who has helped with my children, our business, and keeping our home in happy order in many more ways than I can list. Thank you, Elisa, for being part of our family.

Lastly, I would like to thank my family. Thanks to my daughters, who help me cook and shop and test recipes and who are honest in their opinions, ALWAYS. I enjoy the spirit and spunk of my daughters, who have kept me energetic through the writing and developing of this program. Thank you to my husband for always being there for me, for offering support, and for loving me no matter what. Jason, you are my true soul mate and I am grateful to have you, Sadie, and Zienna as part of my existence.

PART 1

What Is Affecting Health Today?

To keep the body in good health is a duty . . .
otherwise we shall not be able to keep
our mind strong and clear.

—BUDDHA

CHAPTER 1

The True Definition of Health

The idea of optimal health has morphed significantly over time. What we thought was healthy twenty years ago may not be thought of as healthy now. What we thought was unhealthy twenty years ago may be the newest health fad of today. How do you navigate the worlds of health care and diet? With the abundance of information on the Internet and the unending new diet books on the market, how do you decide what is right for you? It can be confusing and daunting to pick the right program. My answer to this confusion is that it is no longer okay to sit and do nothing. Picking any one of the many health diets out there is most likely more helpful to your health than continuing to eat the way you do currently. Making no decision is the worst decision. So I am proud of you for reading this and am excited about your future health changes.

Paradigms of health care are changing constantly. I believe in improved body physiology, which means the body is working better and has improved daily functions. To be truly healthy means to be completely healthy internally. Health is not based on the fact that you lack the symptom today that you had yesterday. Taking a pharmaceutical drug to ward off symptoms is no longer the best answer to health issues and, frankly, never was. The aware and educated patients I see in my office are beginning to question the catch-all use of pharmaceutical medications. Pharmaceutical medications are oftentimes not desired and even rejected by many people in society today. Patients are beginning to truly understand the implications that occur when we Band-Aid symptoms. The symptoms that were masked will return or worsen once the pharmaceutical medications are discontinued. People are demanding a different paradigm of health care now. They want to be involved, they want to work, and they want to heal. And when patients heal, they improve their current and future health.

It is no longer okay to merely suppress symptoms. When we suppress symptoms, we are prolonging the causative health issue and resulting symptoms. Over time, the longer you suppress symptoms, the more difficult it can be to reverse the disease process. Patients don't want their symptoms suppressed; they want their bodies to heal. And remember, when people heal, over time, symptoms improve.

When reversing the disease process, it is important to think about making the body function better. When the body functions better, we should see disease reversal. Most importantly, improving cellular function, especially of the elimination organs, is how we start the best foundation for disease reversal. When you are able to eliminate properly, you are less likely to put your overload into disease states.

Health and the body are beautiful, and I believe that nothing our body does is by accident. Everything the body does, even a symptom, is to survive longer in its environment. So, for example, creating a cancerous tumor in the body is the body's way of walling off and storing a problem so that the body can survive longer. If a person's body were to allow the problem it was originally facing to continue on without trying to combat it and keep it at bay, then they may die within days. But sometimes, when the body is able to wall off this overactive process, a person can live for 20 years beyond the first mutation of the cells. Although cancer poses its own problems, to the body, this was the best option for survival.

Also, the idea of health can be related to your perspective of your body. The more positive one can stay with one's thoughts and visual images of health, the more likely one is to stay that way for a longer period of time. If someone's mental and emotional health is not good, even if his or her body is healthy, his or her view of themself can significantly affect the body's day-to-day health and future risks for illness.

The Importance of Diet

Adopting a healthy, balanced diet can begin to eliminate many of the problems associated with waste accumulation in the body. It also provides adequate nutrients essential to the body's balanced equilibrium. The role of the digestive system is to bring food in, break it down into useable energy via nutrient absorption, and dispose of wastes that cannot be efficiently used. The higher the quality of food we eat, the more nutrients and energy we obtain from it and the less waste burden our body needs to process.

Mitigating the Effects of Poor Diet Overload

We are exposed daily to both environmental toxins and food byproducts accumulated through diet. As we ingest nonuseable chemicals contained in foods, such as hormones, pesticides, antibiotic residues, and other compounds, our body must work extra hard to digest these foreign substances in addition to obtaining nutrients from the same foods. The liver and kidneys, which are responsible for metabolizing compounds, must work at breaking down chemicals and compounds from our environment, our food, and our own metabolic processes. The human body is not 100 percent efficient as it performs metabolism, especially when overburdened by foreign compounds. The body can make excess waste, endogenous material that needs to be processed and excreted from the body. Everyone inherits a different ability for metabolism and storage of waste material. The efficiency with which a person's body excretes these cumulative wastes determines his or her "terrain," the body's susceptibility to disease due to its biochemical and energetic environment. As this implies, different individuals have different terrains.

In addition to environmental and dietary toxins, pharmaceutical drugs or recreational drugs are another source of body burden. Again, the liver and kidneys are mainly responsible for catabolizing (breaking down) and either excreting or storing these toxins. Storing is not the best solution for the body to choose for some of these compounds and chemicals, but when the compounds are new in our environment and foreign to the body, such as some man-made chemicals are, some people's metabolic actions simply cannot tolerate the new chemical. Thus, it is stored away in the body "somewhere safe." Examples of areas where your body might store excess burden may be growths, tumors, fat tissue, fibroid tissue, cholesterol, liver, and nervous system tissue found in nerves, joints, and various other places. I use the term "somewhat safe" because the body has an innate intelligence that chooses storage places in the body that are not vital to your immediate survival, but will affect your long-term health. You can imagine, over time, if we continue to store what we don't understand, we accumulate a total body burden that precedes chronic illness. Some individuals are better at excreting waste, and some individuals like to package and store. This is mainly based on genetics and the environment people grew up in. Those who excrete well are usually healthier individuals but may experience more acute reactions and skin reactions.

Finally, in addition to having to metabolize waste, the body must be able to digest and break down airborne and food-borne allergens. Does it make sense to overload our systems by accumulating more total body burden? What makes sense is reducing dietary toxins, additives, and unnecessary chemicals so we can enhance how effectively we eliminate the remaining ones.

The Cup Analogy

I like to think about everyone having a particular capacity to take things without overflowing. Everyone has a limit. Everyone has a particular set of consequences that add up to exhibiting symptoms. This "cup," as I call it, is a symbol of how much a person can take in. Your cup begins filling at birth. First you must put in your genetic inheritance from your mom's side and then add to it the genetic inheritance from your dad's side. Then comes birth trauma or any issues that occur after birth that affect your growth and development. For example, not being breastfed and being born early or via C-section can all add to your cup. Then the cup is also filled with environmental toxins that you are exposed to from birth and that accumulate over time. Any stressors that you experience throughout your lifetime, including lack of sleep, times in your life when you partied too much and didn't sleep enough, or studied too much and didn't sleep enough, go into your cup. Then you add to this aging, when your body isn't doing things as quickly as it used to and can't adjust as fast as it did when you were in your 20s. Additionally, you fill your cup with stressors such as accidents, relationship stress, school stress, work stress, family stress, financial stress, and so on.

At some point in this accumulation, the cup can overflow, and this is when we see symptoms. Anyone starting from the point of having inherited strong negative genetic susceptibilities may overflow their cup sooner than average and exhibit symptoms sooner than you would expect. Additionally, when someone has pretty strong positive genetics, they seem to be more resilient compared with the average person and are able to vary more from healthy habits and still remain in relative good health. The way the "cup"—your body—empties or drains is through the use of elimination organs. When elimination is efficient, additional accumulation issues are kept from overflowing. The important organs that keep us healthy by continuing to drain the cup are our kidneys, liver, gastrointestinal tract, and the smaller organs associated with these systems. If the function of those elimination organs is clogged or sluggish, then we see our body trying to figure out a different way to remove toxins, such as through the lungs or skin, hence asthma or eczema, or the cup overflows and we see symptoms.

Because of the body's intelligence, we may be aware that the elimination organs are not working efficiently, even though there are no external symptoms. This may present as a serious situation later; when we can't use our elimination organs and genetically we are not prone to asthma or eczema, the issues sometimes travel deeper into the body, forming growths, going into joints, fatty liver, adipose tissue, and so on. This is this person who has been steadily going along in life with no significant issues and then is all of a sudden diagnosed with cancer.

So, when I think of optimal health, I think first of the elimination organs. They are central to your health and central to healing disease. Anyone wanting to reverse disease of any kind must pay special attention to these elimination organs because as they function better, the cup overflows less. There are many ways we can increase the function of our elimination organs, but some of the simplest ways are best. For example, to ensure that our kidneys are functioning optimally, we may simply drink enough clean filtered water every day to ensure we are flushing the right toxins out of that route of elimination. To make sure that our gastrointestinal tract is functioning optimally, we may simply consume a large amount of vegetables, ensuring enough fiber for adequate elimination through bowel movements. And lastly, to help the liver function better, we may avoid excess toxicity such as chemicals in cleaning products, perfumes, and lotions, as well as food items that are difficult for the liver to process, such as alcohol, food additives, sugar, and fried foods. Additionally, understanding the implications and risk for harm that poly-pharmacy causes on the liver is important. Many people are put on too many pharmaceutical medications, and the liver must process these in addition to nearly everything else we put into our bodies.

Another way to conceptualize this analogy is to think about it like this. If you fill the cup with six ounces of poor food choices, stress, genetic susceptibilities, and other chemicals, in addition to your daily metabolism load, you can take in only two more ounces before the cup overflows and you can no longer deal with the excess. If you are then exposed to environmental toxins, pollens in the springtime, and pharmaceutical drugs, your cup cannot handle all the insults to your system. As your cup overflows, you may experience pain, runny nose, postnasal drip, cough, rash, fatigue, anxiety, high blood pressure, and elevated cholesterol, among a myriad of other symptoms.

On the other hand, if you remove the four to six ounces of irritant foods and excess chemicals, you have an increased ability to take in more and process environmental compounds and allergens that cannot be avoided in your daily life. For example, patients who are extremely allergic to grass and pollen cannot remove all the grass and pollen from their lives, but they can decrease their inflammatory foods and additives to allow their body to better process grass and pollens.

Excess inflammation in the body from any source adds to the burden the body must process, thus increasing how much is in the cup. The more inflammation you have, the more all body processes are clouded, and the more the body has to continue working through the inflammation before it can get back to its regular daily jobs of metabolism. Minimizing inflammatory foods, including harmful sugars, and taking in fewer chemicals and compounds through diet reduce inflammation and improve health, reducing the burden on the body.

The Problems with Our Current Lifestyle Habits

To say it lightly, there are a few hiccups in our current lifestyle habits as Western and developed societies. Some of these habits may be easy to change, and some may be so ingrained in the functioning of our society that we may only be able to do our best to minimize our involvement in the health-demoting habit.

I can't say enough how much control you have over your own lifestyle habits. We allow ourselves to get sucked into routines that are not healthful for us. Our work and school schedules can sometimes lead to negative behaviors, causing us to shirk good exercise habits, eat out for lunch too often, not drink enough water, and ultimately increase the amount of stress we feel. And in today's society, who isn't busy? So what I say is look at yourself, look at your schedule, and figure out what you need to do to incorporate better habits. Here's the deal: you will only be around for at most 100 years, or maybe more for a lucky few of you. Make the most of them and exist in the healthiest vessel you can.

Lack of Exercise

For example, one of our main cultural problems is lack of exercise and increasingly sedentary lifestyles. Increased time at work can promote more sedentary habits. Long commutes can leave a person sitting longer and losing the important time they need to add exercise to their daily routine. Driving children around after school and in the evening can lead to parents losing out on their own forms of exercise in order to offer their children opportunities. Parents who don't set a good example of movement and exercise, however, don't teach their children the importance of moving.

According to a meta-analysis published by *Biomed Central Public Health* in 2014, sedentary lifestyle is linked to greater all-cause mortality in older adults. This means sedentary individuals are more likely to be ill and die sooner than those who regularly perform movement or exercise.[1] Another important study by the *British Journal of Sports*

Medicine published in 2011 reported that less time spent sitting was associated with DNA protection and increased telomere length. This is a huge finding because shortened telomere length has been associated with faster aging and increased risk for dementia.[2]

Recently there were two large studies published in the *Journal of the American Medical Association* that support the link between exercise and a significantly reduced risk of premature death.[3] One of the studies revealed that 450 minutes per week of exercise, or a little more than an hour per day, was associated with a 39 percent lower risk of dying prematurely compared to never exercising. And this includes just walking in some cases. This is a HUGE statistic. Now, if over an hour of exercise daily is difficult for you to accomplish, plenty of studies suggest that less than an hour per day is also connected to a lower risk of premature death. The people who did not exercise at all had the largest risk for premature death, so this means that ANYTHING counts.

I can't express enough the importance of exercise. Exercise makes the body know that it is alive and has something to live for. If you are continually moving, then your body feels used and knows it needs to keep up cell regeneration and youthfulness so it can continue the movement it was designed for. If you allow your body to sit constantly day after day, then it doesn't know to keep up the health of your spine, muscles, bones, heart for circulation, skin for elimination, and so forth. It is analogous to an inactive car. If you allow a car to sit in a lot day after day and don't use it, the health of the engine and body goes through a slow process of degradation. When you finally want to use it, it may not even start.

Sedentary Behavior Linked to Diabetes

Sedentary behavior is strongly linked to increased risk for developing type 2 diabetes. Exercise aside, daily habits that are more sedentary compared to daily habits that involve a lot of movement are significantly more associated with the development of diabetes. Sedentary behavior is not simply lack of exercise; the behavior often goes much deeper than that. Spending hours on the couch watching TV, not participating in movement such as walking places daily, and sitting a lot or lying down during the day can be detrimental sedentary behaviors that can increase a person's risk for diabetes and other diseases. Sedentary behavior is also linked to obesity, heart disease, PCOS, insulin resistance, poor lipid profiles, and premature mortality.

Exercise for Depression

Our bodies were not meant to sit as much as we do. Our physical brain needs stimulation, and the way that we do that is through exercise and movement. If we don't continue to stimulate the part of our brain wired for physical activity, it no longer gets to participate in the whole-body hormone orchestra. When we exercise, we stimulate the production of important hormones, namely endorphins, which are chemicals that help us feel better. Not exercising is a great way to lower the body's release of endorphins, thus lowering the body's natural way of feeling happier. There are numerous studies supporting exercise for depressed or sad moods. Above and beyond the well-known health benefits of exercise for the physical body and for decreasing chronic disease risk, exercise has a significant impact on emotional disorders. Some of the strongest evidence of exercise benefiting psychiatric wellness is for depression. Some studies have even shown that exercise was as effective as pharmaceutical therapy not only in the treatment of depression, but also in prevention of depression recurrence.

In a recent depression study, a pharmaceutical intervention group of individuals was compared to a group of individuals who were given a specific exercise program.[4] After a 10-month follow-up of the individuals who continued to exercise, they found that the exercise group was significantly less likely to relapse into depression compared to those taking pharmaceutical medications to treat their depression. What this may mean for many people is that exercise may not only have physical benefit, but will also keep them happier for longer. Who doesn't want that? And most of the time, exercise can come cheaply. Now I am not saying that if you are currently taking a pharmaceutical medication for depression you should discontinue it and begin exercising. What I am saying is that even if you are taking pharmaceutical medications for depression, you should still begin a consistent and deliberate exercise program.

Exercise for Chronic Pain

Exercise is the best medicine for many ailments. Studies have revealed that exercise is related to better outcome for patients with chronic pain. Exercising may prove difficult for some patients in pain, but exercises should be altered to fit each chronic pain patient individually. For example, a study presented at the American Academy of Pain Medicine's 24th Annual Meeting revealed that modest exercise at about five hours per week in chronic pain patients provided a statistically significant reduction in anxiety and depressed mood.[5] The research study also suggested that modest exercise for chronic pain patients led to improved mood and physical capability.

Increased Stress

Before diving into the topic of stress, let me help you understand a little bit more about your autonomic nervous system. Your autonomic nervous system is the system that is active all the time performing all the body processes that occur without your conscious effort. It is automatic. This system controls your breathing, hormone balance, sleep, blood pressure, and heartbeat, as well as various other actions the body needs for survival. The autonomic nervous system can be broken into two important systems: the sympathetic system and the parasympathetic system.

The sympathetic system is the system that prepares the body for emergent or stressful situations. We call this the "fight or flight" system. You either fight or you run. The parasympathetic system is the system that is opposite your stress system. It is stimulated during times of rest, is needed for proper digestion, is extremely important in healing and sleep, and is the main system that is alive during sexual relations. It is an important system that helps manage the excess stress we encounter in our daily lives. The parasympathetic system also inhibits many of the body processes stimulated by the sympathetic system. The sympathetic system is usually dominant and is used to regulate many body processes important to survival. It is an important system but needs to be balanced by the parasympathetic system in order to achieve optimal health.

Many people exist in a sympathetic-dominant state due to their extreme life stressors and lack of proper sleep. If we stay sympathetic-dominant through life, chemical pathways of stress will continue to be stimulated and favored. Therefore, we can get addicted to the stress chemicals our body makes just like we can get addicted to caffeine, nicotine, or any other drug. Chemicals that we make in our body stimulate receptors so that stress feels pretty darn good initially. We get all these chemicals that make us feel really alive and useful and alert and ready. But then the stress is not short-lived and continues to be a burden on the body. These initial bursts of stress chemicals and immediate stimulation of the sympathetic system were meant for quick reactions to stressors, such as running from a tiger or getting out of the way of a speeding car. But now our society offers so much stress in the form of deadlines, traffic, busy schedules, tests, relationship stress, financial stress, and so on that our sympathetic system is in overdrive. No one's body can maintain this long-term; therefore, the prolonged imbalance burns out the nervous system.

I could write an entire book about stress and feel like I hadn't given enough information. Simply said, stress and its health effects are the largest detrimental health epidemic that our species has experienced since something like the plague. Only the plague was easier to pinpoint because it killed quickly and the number of casualties was easily calculated. Stress and its likely counterpart, inflammation, kills slowly. Chronically.

Health Detriments from Stress

Stress is an extremely detrimental factor in the development of chronic illness. First of all, the same chemical mediators that are increased when you are under stress are the same chemical stimulators of inflammation. The connection between increased stress and increased inflammation has become progressively clearer. A recent article published in the *American Heart Journal* revealed that increased anger and mental stress are related to a higher incidence of silent ischemia (when oxygen doesn't get to the heart muscles properly).[6] Numerous studies have connected stress to increased risk for heart disease and heart attack.

But who's to say that elevated stress and the resulting cortisol imbalance are not affecting us right now? Actually, they are impacting many people. Look at how many people have abdominal obesity, which is directly related to excess stress and excess cortisol and sugar dysregulation, not to mention their increased risk for diabetes and heart disease. The next time you are out and about, start counting; the number will shock you.

In addition, how many people do you hear talking about feeling tired and fatigued? This is most likely a result of adrenal burnout or adrenal dysfunction. The adrenal glands are small glands that sit on top of the kidneys. One of their main jobs is to secrete stress hormones such as cortisol. I sometimes refer to them as your body's energy glands. How many people are drinking soda or coffee or newly marketed "energy drinks" daily to increase their energy or performance at work? They need the caffeine and, in most cases, sugar to survive because their own metabolism is out of balance, most likely due to their adrenals. Scarier is that many teenagers are drinking these energy drinks to increase their athletic performance. A recent study revealed that 8.8 percent of all beverages consumed by high school students are energy drinks.[7] These energy drinks are high in caffeine and can be harmful for children to consume. In addition, the size of these drinks is increasing, and although they may list on the bottle that it contains two or three servings, there is no way of sealing the can back up, so it gets consumed all in one serving.

Cortisol is the hormone that is supposed to wake us up in the morning and help us start our days. If we abuse it, overuse it, and disrupt its regular metabolism, we're going to feel out of whack. I often call the problem that occurs with many people's energy "wired and tired." Many of my patients don't have energy during the day but then they are a bit anxious and can't sleep at night. Their bodies have lost the ability to regulate. They can't get back into a balanced, normal circadian rhythm with increased levels of stress affecting their energy gland's function.

In modern life stress starts young! Very young for some children, as they might be struggling with abusive parents, absent parents, or drug-affected parents. Often young children are put under more and more pressure to perform, succeed, compete with other children, and so on. I can attest to these changes even in my own children, who are six years apart. The school agenda items that my younger daughter is tackling now are the same things my older daughter might have been assigned one grade higher. I remember my first daughter doing a lot of playing and art in kindergarten, and when my younger daughter was in kindergarten, only six years later, there was a lot less playing and drawing and a lot more focus on reading and math skills.

Stress at a young age can even affect cortisol levels years later. Cortisol is the hormone connected to the stress response, but it also plays a major role in regulating blood glucose. Originally this important stress response was needed by our species back in hunter-and-gatherer times because we needed to be able to move quickly to run from a predator or to catch our prey. When stress hormones increase, our body naturally increases blood sugar for those quick bursts. But the reality is that we have a significant amount of stress coupled with a significant number of sedentary habits, and this is not a good combination. So when a person is under a lot of stress, regardless of age, their cortisol levels increase, thereby increasing their glucose levels. If stress is maintained for a long period of time, then so is blood glucose. Higher levels of blood glucose over time can worsen insulin sensitivity and promote diabetes in later life. A prolonged higher level of glucose also leads to increased oxidative stress and advanced and premature aging.

Interestingly, a recent study of over 100 at-risk young children revealed that those who were put into a 10-week-long nurturing, loving program had improved cortisol levels even three years later, again proving that elevated stress and cortisol levels experienced as young children can affect future cortisol balance.[8]

Increased family stress can have a huge detriment on the behavior of children as they go through adolescence. Oftentimes, families are no longer sitting down together to enjoy each other's company. Children have sports, parents work late, and a multitude of events are scheduled. The family that spends time together has healthier, balanced children. Studies have revealed that a lack of family sit-down dinners predicts higher risk for behaviors such as alcohol and drug use in older children.

Increased daily living expenses and college loans, home loans, and car loans have pushed our society to adopt the two-working-parent household in many homes. This can provide more financial comfort, but it does present some interesting dilemmas. Is someone cooking nourishing foods, or is the family eating out, carrying in, or eating processed foods? Is someone helping the children with their homework, or is the child finding the answers online? Who is teaching the children how to live their lives by the example that they are presenting? If your child sees you always running around from thing to thing, minute to minute, they often will adopt these behaviors in their lives. I see numerous young teenagers in my office feeling extreme pressure and stress from school: deadlines, papers, sports, etc. Now, I am not saying that you quit everything, throw in the towel, and walk into the woods to live out your life in seclusion. I am just saying you should pay attention to the balance you are creating for your family and others who live near and around you.

Meditation for Health

In a study published in *The Journal of the American Medical Association* in February of 2015, meditation was connected with improved sleep, less fatigue, and improved depression. The study took two groups. One was given sleep hygiene tips and the other was given meditation. The mindfulness meditation helped people in this group have better sleep and less daytime fatigue and fewer feelings of depression compared with their counterpart group.[9]

A significant number of recent studies show how meditation can improve day-to-day quality of life in addition to reducing a number of health ailments. For example, you can find positive meditation studies demonstrating help with migraines, pain, anxiety, depression, memory, reducing aging, Alzheimer's prevention, and more. We will discuss a simple meditation technique in Chapter 10.

Another new study conducted by Morehouse Medical School and Emory University assigned a year-long meditation program to African Americans to see what kind of effect it would have on endothelial (blood vessel) health. The study showed that there was a significant improvement in endothelial function. Along with that, those who were randomly assigned to the year-long meditation program showed improvements in blood pressure, weight, and triglycerides. [10]

More Media Means New Issues

The combination of more media, easier access to the Internet, and numerous phone apps has increased the likelihood of a sedentary lifestyle. Many jobs that were once done outside can now be done on the computer. More computer work means less movement and increased sitting. I am standing up right now at my bar moving my legs because I have been sitting here too long writing. I am going to take a break to exercise. If you are not lying in bed reading this, take a 10-minute break and do some movement. Move in place, do some jumping jacks, do some stretching, walk up and down your stairs, then come back to reading and you will feel a bit more energized.

More media means a lot of other things, too. For one thing, it means less eye contact. The more we reduce our direct contact with people and choose to communicate through media resources, the less connected we can feel, and this will affect our health. Feeling connected and having a purpose are what help us survive and want to continue surviving in this world. Even the Framingham heart study that was performed in the 1950s found that the lack of a significant other and of connection with others increases risk for heart disease.[11,12]

Again, more media means that everyone in the house has his or her own device. Family members no longer have to sit together in the evenings to enjoy eating dinner, watching TV, or doing anything else together. Children are playing with their iPads while parents are checking their email and the dog is listening to his iPod. (Just kidding.)

Children are learning their social and emotional interactions through media. Consider that with media, they may not know how to develop their own emotions and reactions to circumstances that occur in their lives because they have seen everything before. Media has shown them how to react to everything—their dad dies, thier cat dies, they flunk a test, they experience a break-up—and, additionally, it has taught them how to react to their parents' problems. Parents get divorced, they lose a job . . . we have seen it all in the movies, and we have seen how people react, and it is with a lot of drama. No TV show reflects healthy individuals dealing with their stressors in a less-than-dramatic way. Let's face it; drama sells movies and television shows, and that is how our young ones are learning their face-to-face contact with people and difficult situations. Similarly, this is why bullying in schools has increasingly become a problem. Many shows cast a dominant character who takes advantage of a weaker or younger character.

For children, experiencing life through the lens of heightened drama increases stress. Young children are learning to experience their world as a series of stressful challenges rather than learning to face their world as a series of opportunistic challenges that teach and show them how to grow and mature. Then as adults, it is easy to carry this drama into our workplace, our homes, our relationships, and so forth.

Additionally many children are allowed to take media, such as an iPad or their phones, to bed, which causes them to get less sleep. For example, just having that phone in bed with them at night can cause them to be on it longer than if they didn't have it in bed with them. Children will offer many excuses such as, "But I need it for my alarm." So get them an alarm clock and move the media out of the bedroom. Not to mention that removing the electromagnetic waves from the bedroom at night will also promote better sleep.

More Social Media Means More Pressure

Social media is at the height of popularity for most generations, from adolescents to adults. Virtual social spaces are created by the many social media applications that we have access to. Virtual social spaces can be where young children and adults feel their worth. How many likes did you get on that picture? How much are you worried about the fact that your comment or picture didn't get any likes? There are great studies demonstrating an elevation in dopamine levels when study subjects received a text or a "like" on the picture they just uploaded onto social media. Having yourself and your personal information on social media means that everyone now has the potential to be a public figure. This is a lot of pressure for the younger generation and can also be a lot of pressure for adults. Having to compete now in an additional way adds to the stress of daily life. Then if you have to maintain the many social networks, you or your children may be under even more stress to "keep up" socially. Have I looked at my

Instagram or Facebook lately? Am I going to be out of the loop if I don't get on it daily and like everyone's photos? I am speaking from experience here with my adolescent at home. We can't deny them the use of social media, but we can certainly be a bit smarter about time limits and when they are allowed access.

We have to remember that we have an extreme power in our hands with the use of computers, phones, and other electronic devices. We can make messages that have the potential to reach far and wide. We can make a video that goes viral. We can post something that thousands of people can see within seconds. With that power comes stress. Now we are no longer competing only with our small and immediate peer group; we are competing with peer groups from all over the world. Young adults and adolescents have an extreme pressure to perform in their virtual social worlds.

More Media Means No White Space

Do you remember being bored when you were young? Yes, you had to just sit there and think about what you should do. Sometimes when you were waiting for someone to come over, you might have daydreamed a little bit. Used your imagination. Interestingly enough, we don't really get to experience that "white space" anymore. Even adults who grew up with white space don't know what to do with themselves when they are sitting at a stoplight, waiting in line, or waiting for anything for that matter. Look around, you see it all the time. People don't know what to do with themselves if they are not able to look down at their phones when they have even the shortest empty moment. I believe this is causing us to lose a little bit of our creativity. Our calm. Our time to reset or just breathe.

I believe that when we are able to have a little white space in our lives, we can combat burnout. When we run from activity to activity without any time for rest in between, sometimes our whole day can be encompassed by fast-paced, stressful deadlines. White spaces, even little ones when you take a deep breath and don't look at your phone, help create a small stimulation of your parasympathetic system.

I discussed meditation a little earlier. Meditation doesn't always have to be the sit-down type you are thinking of. Sometimes just taking a small amount of time to calm yourself and relax can be meditative for the body. As discussed earlier, there are ample studies supporting the use of meditation for improving health. Meditation has been shown to decrease blood pressure and cardiac risk as well as reduce anxiety, depression, and anger. Specifically, it reduces risk for Alzheimer's disease because it helps the brain chemicals function more appropriately, aiding the communication between different parts of the brain.

So try this. The next time you are sitting anywhere you would normally grab for your phone, don't. Just close your eyes for a second and breathe, and allow your mind to wander like it used to.

Lack of Sleep

I always discuss sleeping habits with my patients. When we sleep we heal. Sleep is crucial to your overall health, and it is difficult to pinpoint everything that is occurring in your body while you sleep. There are thousands of processes that are occurring at night while you sleep, rebooting your system for the next day. The body detoxes while sleeping and the skeletal muscles get to rest. The liver processes toxicity, and hormones are made and broken down.

Many studies have connected poor sleep to worse health and performance outcomes. A recent study conducted on medical school residents found that those who didn't sleep as much due to working more hours were more fatigued and made more medical errors than those who slept more hours.[13] And according to a report published in 2013, medical errors in the United States were the third leading cause of death. This research estimated that up to 440,000 Americans are dying annually from preventable hospital errors.[14] Many of these errors could be occurring because of doctors and nurses who are working long hours and are sleep-deprived.

A large US study that has followed patients for years has found that less sleep (less than seven hours nightly) is related to higher heart disease risk in those who are obese or overweight. This study has also shown that patients who have four specific risk factors have significantly higher all-cause mortality, including higher rates of cardiovascular disease and cancer. The four risk factors are low sleep (less than seven hours per day), low exercise (less than one hour per week), high TV viewing (greater than three hours per day), and overweight (BMI greater than 25).[15]

Seconding the previous study, according to the National Institutes of Health, everyone should be getting more than seven hours of sleep to ward off high blood pressure, diabetes, depression, obesity, and cancer.

Sleep is important in controlling many functions in the body, including the immune system, balancing hormones, memory and learning, as well as weight loss. When you sleep is when you repair. One of the most important mechanisms of repair that occurs at night while you are sleeping is keeping your blood vessels healthy. Considering that heart disease is still the number-one killer of both men and women in the United States, I would consider putting more emphasis on how much you sleep at night.

Many of you may be thinking that you don't have to worry about repairing your blood vessels because you don't have heart disease, and many of you already understand your heart health. Either way, you should listen up. Many times, especially in women, the very first cardiovascular symptom someone experiences is death. This situation doesn't offer much leniency to make changes for the future. So make them now, because like it or not, you may already have arterial damage and blockages that could be putting you at risk for heart disease.

I cannot stress enough the importance of sleep for maintanence of cognitive function, improved mood, better energy, and decreased risk for chronic illness. Additionally, any weight loss program should include getting eight hours of sleep per night. If this seems absurd to you, then maybe it is time to figure out how to get yourself to sleep better. I have suggestions listed at the end of the book.

Dietary Imbalances

Let's talk about what the diet is like now compared to what the diet used to be like 50 years ago, 100 years ago, and before. It's interesting that 50 years ago, some of our most detrimental dietary trends were introduced. As early as the late 1800s, trans fats were introduced into the food industry, and they began being used in foods around the 1910s, namely in items such as Oreo cookies and Crisco. Yes, they were available that early on.

Food-Processing Revolution Was Not a Health Revolution

World War I brought about more food processing to make cooking easier. This is when we started to see more processed foods available, such as canned items and frozen foods. Processed food advertisements promised to save time for housewives. Some foods available after WWI were condiments, Wonder Bread, Kool-Aid, and Peter Pan Peanut Butter. Then in the 1930s, depressed times called for money-tightening strategies and cutbacks on the types of foods purchased. With the Great Depression beginning, families had to get by on less. In the 1930s, Snickers candy bars, Kraft Macaroni & Cheese, and Ritz Crackers were highlights of the processed foods consumed.

After the 1930s, the availability of products that contained processed foods and hydrogenated oils increased greatly. Food advertisements continued to promote the quality, flavor, and ease of use and preparation of processed foods over foods made from scratch. This is when we really started to take a turn for the worse in our food options. Many items from this time on were produced with trans fats, also referred to as "hydrogenated oils" on food labels. The processed foods becoming available during this time contained an increasing amount of dehydrated food items, such as the powdered cheese in macaroni and cheese.

Then another war hit in the 1940s, the Second World War. Due to low rations and many men being drafted, the household income dropped dramatically. Women who had never worked before were forced to pick up jobs that were low paying just to try and make ends meet. In addition, food rations needed to be sent to the soldiers; therefore we experienced the development of yet more processed foods that would not spoil. This is when we saw an increase in "convenience" foods such as instant coffee, dehydrated juice, frozen foods, and baked good mixes. The first Dairy Queen and McDonald's restaurants opened, offering quick, cheap, easy meals. Government subsidies were created to promote corn and soy use, which resulted in the increased use of high-fructose corn syrup, hydrogenated oils, and other processed foods. The highlight of the 1940s and 1950s was convenience cooking and living.

High-Fructose Corn Syrup

One of the most detrimental foods ever introduced into our food supply is high-fructose corn syrup. We will discuss later the formation and consumption of advanced glycation end products (AGEs), compounds that are detrimental to overall health by promoting conditions including diabetes and aging progression, but for now note that fructose more readily forms these dangerous compounds than any other sugar. Our diets contained excessive amounts of high-fructose corn syrup from the 1940s or 1950s until at least the 2000s, and you can still find many products that primarily contain high-fructose corn syrup. There are many families still purchasing these products and, by doing so, increasing their children's risk for diabetes and other chronic health complaints.

Here are some food items that most likely still contain high-fructose corn syrup:

- juices that are not 100 percent juice
- sodas
- chilled, flavored drinks, such as tea and energy drinks
- breakfast cereal, especially popular name brands
- yogurt
- salad dressings
- condiments such as ketchup, mayonnaise, mustard, and relish
- breads
- baked goods
- candy and candy bars
- nutrition or protein bars
- granola bars
- infant formulas (contain corn-syrup solids)

Make sure when you are following this program, once you begin to introduce foods back into your diet, that you pay special attention to all food labels. Some items will surprise you.

Overconsumption of Sugar

One ever-pressing problem with the standard diet of today's world is that we have all grown accustomed to consuming way too much sugar. Sugar permeates almost every meal now unless you make an effort to avoid it. Most morning breakfasts are centered on a sweet and satisfying taste. When I suggest to my patients to have a salad for breakfast or sauté some zucchini, they really think the recommendation is absurd.

Overconsumption of sugar burns out the pancreas and the liver because they work in unison to maintain healthy, balanced blood sugar levels. It also leads to overweight children and sometimes obesity in adults, as well as improper insulin response and insulin resistance. Sure, if you are not type 1 diabetic, you can eat loads of sugar all through childhood and not suffer the effects. But if you look at the trend for developing type 2 diabetes today, you will be astonished. If we can work toward better balance for children, we can do a better job of preventing type 2 diabetes later on in life. Diabetes will be discussed in future chapters.

When you consume sugar, you are allowing your body to get full on "empty" calories, and then you're not hungry for and don't have a taste for the most important foods, like vegetables.

Also, when you consume sugary foods that lack fiber and protein, the blood sugar spikes. This feels great at first, almost like a high, but then the blood sugar drops quickly and radically because you have sequestered so much insulin to remove the sugar from the blood and into the cells. When this occurs, you find yourself ravenously hungry. When you eat fiber and vegetables instead, you experience a slow, steady rise in blood sugar, a normal insulin response, and a slow, steady uptake of glucose into the cells. When you consume a high-sugar diet, the body regularly gets bombarded with too much sugar. Then postmeal, when the body is still trying to balance the blood sugar, the pancreas and insulin are usually no longer big players. This is when your body has to decide how to store this excess "energy," or extra calories brought into the body. How the body wants to deal with this, if it is functioning well and is balanced, is to store this excess as glycogen in the liver. The glycogen can be easily accessed later and broken back down into blood sugar so that the body can enjoy the balance. With prolonged excess energy problems, along with improper nutrition to facilitate optimal function, the body is no longer able to efficiently store blood sugar when there is excess. When this occurs, we see the body begin to favor storage as fat. And when we begin to store as fat, this process is difficult to reverse without a drastic dietary change.

I believe this biochemical imbalance in the body is why so many people diet but cannot lose weight, or they diet and lose weight but cannot keep it off. The biochemistry is still not in balance, and they are still favoring the fat-storage pathway. I believe that one way we can begin to change this is to eat almost no sugar for at least 60 days while consuming almost all vegetables and some protein, like the Freedom Diet suggests. It is surprising how much we are able to switch one process off and one process on with just the proper balance of a vegetable-rich diet.

World Health Organization Recommendation

Recently the World Health Organization researched the sugar intake in various regions of the world and found that in North and Central America, we are consuming upwards of 95 grams of sugar daily on average. In addition, South Americans are consuming about 130 grams and Western Europeans are consuming about 101 grams. Their recommendation as of 2015 is to cut that amount to 50 grams or less. This would account for about 10 percent of people's daily energy intake. Even better, the researchers in the study suggested, would be to decrease sugar consumption to about 5 percent of daily energy intake.[16] Of special note, one sugar-sweetened can of soda contains 40 grams of sugar and one cup of 2 percent milk contains a little over 12 grams of sugar. These numbers add up quickly.

On average, if we think about grams of sugar in terms of teaspoons, Americans are consuming around 23-24 teaspoons of sugar daily. This adds up to over 70 pounds of sugar per year, an astronomical number. Shockingly, American teens are consuming upwards of 34 teaspoons daily. Unfortunately, our overconsumption of sugar is leading to weight gain and obesity, high blood pressure, diabetes, and high cholesterol. Don't forget that morbidity and mortality increase proportionally to someone's weight. Therefore a 400-pound person will have significantly more health risks than a 200-pound person.

American Heart Association Recommendation

The American Heart Association is worried about the sugar consumption in our society and what it will do to our future health as a nation. They have set the following recommendations, which most people are already exceeding. Notice that the recommendation is lowest for children, and also of special note is that teenagers should not be consuming more sugar than their parents.

The sugar consumption recommendations are:

- Children: Limit to 3-4 teaspoons per day
- Adult women/teens: Limit to 5 teaspoons per day
- Adult men/teens: Limit to 8-9 teaspoons per day[17]

Overconsumption of Sweetened Drinks

Overconsuming sugary drinks has increasingly become a problem. Everywhere you look in stores and vending machines, you find sweetened drinks of all kinds. I believe that sugary drinks have become one of the largest sugar sources in our diet. Large coffee drinks, sweetener in coffee, energy drinks, sodas, juice and juice boxes, sweetened tea, fancy alcoholic drinks, lemonade, you name it. Face it; if it has sugar in it, we want to indulge. Sugar is delicious and makes us feel good initially, so it is hard to refuse.

Starting when our children are young, we allow them to drink juice every morning, juice for lunch, and sometimes a large glass of low-fat milk for dinner. Low-fat milk has a significant amount of sugar. Young infants are given juice in their bottles because they never have cultivated a taste for water. Adults who aren't drinking water in front of their children are doing such a disservice to them.

Overconsumption of sugary drinks is one of the leading causes of obesity in children. And children who start out obese are heading toward an inevitable future of diabetes and heart disease if they do not change now. Sugar is bad for you and sugary drinks are worse. They are worse because they don't have any fiber to combat all the sugar you are putting in your body. If you eat a Snickers bar, you at least have fiber and nuts to slow down the blood sugar spike. A study recently conducted in the United Kingdom of 25,000 people found that reducing intake of sugary drinks, sodas, or artificially sweetened drinks was connected to a 14 to 25 percent lower risk of type 2 diabetes. The study also found that drinking artificially sweetened drinks was not connected to a lower risk of diabetes. The study recommended drinking unsweetened drinks as the best option. Replacing even one sweetened drink with unsweetened coffee, water, or tea provided benefits for reducing diabetes risk.[18]

Soda is one of the worst food items we can include in our diets. One can contains double the daily dose of sugar recommended for an adult, according to the American Heart Association. Even worse, many children are consuming soda daily, and in the process ingesting a whopping three times the amount of their recommended daily sugar intake. And this occurs in one sitting. What is the child going to consume for the rest of the day? I am positive that most children who are consuming sodas regularly are also including sugar in other parts of their diets.

Even one soda per day can increase someone's risk for cardiovascular disease by up to 30 percent, and this connection was found independent of other risk factors like obesity and total daily calories.[19] Soda has also been linked to increased aggression in children as well as inattention. Interestingly, the symptoms appeared to be dose dependent. For example, as soda consumption increased in these children, their aggression and inattention worsened.[20]

Below is the sugar content of soda measured in teaspoons:

- 12-ounce can = 10 teaspoons of sugar
- 20-ounce bottle = 16 teaspoons of sugar
- 2-liter bottle = 27 teaspoons of sugar

I don't understand how we didn't know in the 1940s and beyond that corn syrup and sugar are bad for your health. We understood that it was bad for your teeth, but why didn't we as a society clue in to the detrimental effects of sugar? Why did we and why do we still continue to feed our kids Kool-Aid, Lucky Charms, McDonald's, donuts, cakes, cookies, pastries, and processed foods? Convenience? I think that ship has sailed. Time to choose a new path.

Sweet Versus Fake Sweet

What about all the other products out there that are not sweetened with a form of sugar, but are sweetened with a chemical sweetener such as NutraSweet, Sweet'N Low, or Splenda? There are quite a few things wrong with using an unnatural sweetener. Number one, it is an artificial chemical and can have potentially dangerous effects in the body.

Another concern of mine is what happens to the sugar–insulin response that your body is used to stimulating when you consume something sweet. Normally, you take sugar in, your body increases insulin, which allows for you to get the sugar from the bloodstream and into the cell. Easy peasy, right? Well, artificial sweeteners activate sweet taste receptors in enteroendocrine cells, thus causing the release of incretin, a hormone that is known to contribute to glucose absorption. In 2008, both the journals *Circulation* and *Obesity* reported a connection between diet-soda consumption and the development of obesity and metabolic syndrome.[21] Metabolic syndrome will be discussed in more detail later. Additionally, in 2009, it was presented at the 91st annual meeting of the Endocrine Society that people who used artificial sweeteners were twice as likely to develop diabetes compared to those who did not. Those using artificial sweeteners were also more likely to be insulin resistant compared to nonusers.

Back to talking about that sweet taste in your mouth. I have always had concern that the sweet taste of food stimulates an insulin response, but then there is no increased sugar in the bloodstream for your body to metabolize. Then you are stuck with elevated insulin in the bloodstream that has no use. Prolonged consumption of these artificial sweeteners and the consequentially prolonged elevated insulin in the bloodstream will build insulin resistance. The body will no longer stay as sensitive to the insulin as it should be. According to an article published online in September of 2014 in *Nature*, artificial sweeteners such as aspartame, sucralose, and saccharine are directly linked to glucose intolerance.[22] What this means is the regular metabolism of sugar is being altered by the continued consumption of these "fake sugar" foods. It is presumptuous of me to tell you that all artificial sugars act the same way in the body, but there are reasons for concern and caution when choosing your "sweet" food items. I bring this up because it is extremely important information to understand when you are faced with trying to lose weight, improve blood sugar levels, and generate better diet habits. Many of my diabetic patients truly believe they are doing something good for their bodies when they choose "sugar-free" candy or a "sugar-free" diabetic meal-replacement drink.

What is even more interesting is that this study revealed that the glucose control issue began to alter the gut microbiota of the mice that were in the experiment consuming the artificial sweetener. This brings into light an entirely different issue. The gastrointestinal tract is the organ that takes the largest hit when someone consumes an unhealthy diet. The unnatural foods or heavily sugared foods enter through the mouth and are encountered by the gut first. We will discuss more about gastrointestinal health in the next chapter.

Another study published in *Diabetes Care* in 2013 supported the fact that artificial sweeteners wreak havoc on blood sugar balance. Researchers from Washington School of Medicine in St. Louis found that consuming the artificial sweetener Splenda caused large spikes in blood sugar levels after consumption. Additionally, insulin levels on average spiked 20 percent higher than normal, suggesting that regularly consuming artificial sweeteners can increase the risk of insulin resistance.[23]

Artificially sweetened foods and beverages have become a large market, touted as safe for the society and safe for diabetics, but emerging research is suggesting the opposite. So what I say to this is we should always go back to the roots of our food sources. Eat whole foods, don't eat chemically derived foods, don't eat unnatural foods, and don't eat anything that is processed, as the processing itself will be detrimental to the nutrition content of the food and most likely the sugar content of the food.

Glycemic Index

Glycemic index (GI) measures a food's impact on blood sugar (glucose) levels. The higher a food's GI, the more elevated your blood sugar will become as a result of consuming that food. High-GI foods tend to be high in carbohydrates without the benefit of also being high in bulk, fiber, or nutrients. They are typically packed with sugar and calories. The diet today is largely weighted toward high-GI foods that can be harmful to blood sugar balance and future ability to maintain control of the blood sugar with optimal insulin levels. Regularly consuming such foods will result in abnormally elevated glucose levels, which can lead to metabolic issues, weight gain, insulin resistance, and type 2 diabetes. The body is not meant to withstand a continued elevation in glucose.

Over time, consistently elevated glucose negatively impacts lipid levels, triglyceride levels, and inflammation levels. It leads to insulin resistance, weight gain, elevated blood pressure, poor mood, and disrupted sleep. For a table listing the glycemic index for many common foods, please visit *www.glycemicindex.com*. The general rule for good dietary practice is to avoid all high-GI foods, considered to be anything with a rating of 70 or over. Consume only in moderation foods with a medium glycemic index, from 56 to 69. Eat generously all low-GI foods (55 or below). Low-GI foods control appetite better, facilitate weight loss, and reduce inflammation by reducing blood glucose levels. When you are first staring the Freedom Diet, please pay special attention to this, as the more lower-GI foods you consume, the better you will begin to control your blood sugar and facilitate weight loss. In addition, packing your diet full of low-GI foods will increase your satiety, or feeling of fullness, during and after eating.

Know that paying attention to the GI of the foods you eat is only one aspect of decreasing inflammation and improving your health. Just because linguini, for example, fits the bill by being low on the

GI chart doesn't mean that you should indulge in endless servings of linguini. In fact, as you will learn later in the chapter, the Freedom Diet encourages you to avoid eating most grains to ensure the quickest improvement in blood sugar and quality of life.

Underconsumption of Vegetables and Fruits

One large problem with the current diet is that we consume way too many carbohydrates in the form of starches. Breads, pastries, donuts, cereals, cakes, and cookies are overabundant in the diet. They are offered at every social event and are a staple in most homes. Due to the increased consumption of starchy carbohydrates, the real or "good" carbohydrates such as fruits and vegetables are drastically reduced.

According to a review of studies conducted in Europe, Asia, and the United States, consuming more fruits and vegetables decreased the risk for stroke. In fact, stroke risk decreased by 32 percent for every 200-gram increment in daily fruit and vegetable intake.[24] Most individuals do not consume the amount of vegetables they should eat daily. We can all do better by increasing the amount of servings of fresh vegetables per day. This is often a challenge that I give to my patients. Oftentimes for an easy suggestion, I tell my patients to increase their servings of vegetables per day by three. But on the Freedom Diet, I am asking you for something more. Make a larger commitment to your health and transformation.

Ideally when you first start this diet, you should eat seven to eight cups of vegetables per day. This can drastically increase weight loss and improve your body's ability to eliminate waste and balance your blood sugar levels. Consuming this many vegetables may be difficult at first but will feel extremely rewarding after a few weeks. You'll notice your energy and moods start to improve, your blood sugars will stabilize, and you will connect thoughts better in your head. Who doesn't want to be able to think a little bit straighter? If you check your lipid levels before and after commencing this diet, you will be shocked at how much your HDL, the good cholesterol, can increase in addition to your LDL and total cholesterol decreasing. It isn't avoiding fat that brings down your cholesterol; it is eating more vegetables.

Vegetables and fruits offer fiber, better fiber than found in cereals.

Fiber helps with digestion and probiotic balance, and improves food's transit time in the gastrointestinal tract. Probiotics, or "gut bugs," are the healthy bacteria and yeast that inhabit the gastrointestinal lining. Fiber feeds the healthy bacteria and yeast in the GI lining, ensuring their survival. The probiotic lining balance is extremely important in the function of the immune system and is also important in digestion.

Due to many bodily processes being stimulated by the gut, the probiotic balance has been well researched in relation to many conditions, including mental and emotional conditions, metabolism, autoimmune disease, and more. Transit time is important because the amount of time food spends in the GI tract, especially the large and small intestines, is vital to optimal health. When the food sits too long, more toxins can be removed from the food and stored in the body. Conversely, when the food doesn't spend enough time, for example, in the small intestine, it isn't in there long enough for proper nutrient absorption. Additionally, without fiber and proper probiotic balance, you may not have proper predigestion of food, which ensures proper nutrient absorption.

Overconsumption of Gluten

Gluten is the substance in breads, pastries, and other baked goods that is responsible for their elasticity and "gluey" consistency. Gliadin proteins, components of gluten, are a group of proteins found in wheat and other grains that give baked goods the ability to rise in the baking process. The gluten found in wheat has been directly connected to increased weight gain, especially central weight gain. And as I've mentioned, central obesity is directly linked to heart disease.

The overconsumption of gluten is a major problem in the United States. The quality of wheat has changed drastically in the past decades. Due to significant genetic modification, wheat has become a rather hearty crop, less susceptible to the insects and spoilage that once affected it. Now that the crop has become so hearty, we also have a hard time digesting it. For example, wheat grown in this country now has 28 chromosomes instead of its original 14. Now that is a lot of chromosomes! Can you imagine a crop changing that much in 50 years? This new wheat can now code for a significantly greater amount of gluten per serving compared with years ago. Also wheat, especially its component gluten, has the ability to act like a "feel-good" chemical in your body and can be called an exorphin. Similar to an endorphin, exorphins stimulate the same receptors and cause the same feel-good response you crave. Endorphins are released from various mechanisms such as running outside, exercise, receiving exciting news, and even hearing your phone get a text message. Because gluten is an exorphin, guess what? Wheat and all the products that are made with it can become addictive because they give you that happy stimulation. When you eat wheat you are rewarded with happiness.

Now, I am not saying that everyone has a gluten allergy or is gluten intolerant, but what I am saying is that if I can get patients to avoid gluten and baked goods made with gluten flours, the ability to lose weight, improve blood sugar levels, and maintain better mental and emotional health is much easier and quicker. Regularly consuming a lot of gluten inhibits what I am trying to balance with people. It may be that many people are intolerant to gluten due to the balance of the probiotics in their gut lining. As probiotics help us with the digestion of our foods, this proper balance is essential to improved health and improved digestion. Gluten can be a confusing protein for the GI lining to interpret; therefore, removing it can take the burden off the GI lining so it can begin to heal and improve its probiotic balance. I will discuss probiotic balance and its importance in digestion in future chapters.

Uneducated about Fat

It is surprising that not everyone understands the importance of fat in the diet. The "low-fat" diet is one of the diet fads that has lasted the longest in our society. The low-fat diet started its roots in the early 1900s and was popularized in the 1970s. Heart disease has been the leading cause of death among Americans since 1921 and remains the top killer. Stroke was the third-leading cause of death among Americans from 1938 to 2006 and remains the fifth-leading killer in the United States. We have taken strides to reduce these numbers with pharmaceutical medication, reduced rates of smoking, increased exercising, and dietary change. But the fact remains that heart disease is still the number-one killer and the number-one disease we should look to prevent in both men and women.

Our view of dietary fat is beginning to change but is still largely wrong because we keep thinking that fat is the culprit, when really it is more likely that we are not balancing our diet as we should. You have already read about my feelings on the imbalance of the American diet, and all the aspects I have covered so far may lead you to think that fat is the problem. Yes, fat can be the problem if we are not balancing it with plenty of vegetables and a healthy lifestyle.

Unhealthy fats were discussed in depth in my first book, *The Anti-Inflammation Diet and Recipe Book*. What I will repeat here is that we should avoid *all* fried foods and fast foods. Certain frying practices can change the chemical structure of even a healthy cooking oil to produce what is known as a "trans fat." Other names for trans fat are "partially hydrogenated oil" and "partially hydrogenated fat." These unhealthy fats have a direct connection to inflammation, heart disease, and cancer. Our bodies don't utilize this type of fat in any way, so the body tries to incorporate it in some location where it is not vital for survival. For example, we may try to incorporate these unhealthy fats into cell membranes, where they would affect cell membrane function and the transport of important chemicals in and out of cells. Frying and sautéing methods, even at home with healthy oils, can promote the production of unhealthy fats as well. When oils, especially unstable oils such as monounsaturated oils like olive oil, are heated to high heat, this transition to "trans" fatty acids is possible.

When my first book was published, in 2006, there were no laws about labeling foods for trans fat content. But now, the amount of trans fat in a food must be printed on its label. So must the amount of unsaturated fats (the "good" fats) and saturated fats (the so-called "bad" fats). Saturated fats, which come mostly from animal products, including dairy, have also been directly linked to inflammation levels and heart disease. Saturated fats, unlike trans fats, do have a use in the body and, when eaten in moderation in a proper form, can be beneficial.

If you are going to eat animal products, it is much safer to consume organic, grass-fed meat that is free of added hormones and other added chemicals. According to Janet Kim in an interview with Dr. David Katz, health experts are finally realizing that not all saturated fats are created equal. In fact, Dr. Katz brings up an excellent point. We have equally distressing rates of coronary heart disease before and after the removal of saturated fats, accompianied by the introduction of more sugar. Additionally, he makes a second point that we are still struggling with the same health problems even though we have swapped sugar for fat.[25] So is fat the problem or is sugar the problem or is gluten the problem? I have discussed all these issues to emphasize that the overall problem with our diet is not just one thing; rather, it is all the things we are doing wrong combined that increase our risk for illness.

Besides the quality of the saturated fat, it is also important to consider *how much* you consume versus how many vegetables you consume. The most important part of a balanced diet is consuming vegetables. Even a paleo diet can be done right if someone is eating enough vegetables. The problem occurs when we think paleo means eating a lot of fat and protein and making baked goods with ground nut flours and honey.

The Differences in Oils

When using coconut oil (a saturated vegetable fat) or butter for baking, the amount you use is small compared to how much saturated fat you get from eating a steak. One of the benefits of saturated fats is their stability when subjected to the cooking process. A monounsaturated fat like olive oil is less stable and can actually change its chemical structure when overheated, resulting in a trans fat. Don't get me wrong: I love olive oil, and it is one of the three oils I use often in my house, but I rarely heat it, and when I do I use only low to medium-low heat. Coconut oil is largely made up of saturated fatty acids, which are still somewhat controversial because of their link to elevated levels of LDL cholesterol (the bad cholesterol), which in turn have been linked to heart disease. This is why the FDA still doesn't recommend the widespread use of coconut oil. As noted, however, not all saturated fats are necessarily bad for you when consumed in moderation. Research shows that coconut oil has been used by Pacific Island populations for generations, at levels amounting to as much as 30–60 percent of their daily caloric intake, with no evidence of increased heart disease risk. Coconut oil is a very special saturated fat, being one of the few dietary sources of medium-chain fatty acids. Medium-chain fatty acids help boost metabolism and help the body utilize fat for energy, often aiding in weight loss.

One important saturated fatty acid found in coconut oil is lauric acid. Lauric acid, when made into monolaurin in the body, is helpful in boosting the immune system to fight off viruses. I don't have patients consume coconut oil therapeutically during an illness; rather, I have them supplement with either lauric acid or monolaurin. Still, eating coconut oil during an infection is not a bad idea. While there is a general lack of research on the benefits of coconut oil, lauric acid and monolaurin have been shown in the laboratory to have antifungal and antiviral properties. I have used both of them for over ten years for shingles, herpes simplex outbreaks, and influenza with excellent results.

In new research involving animal studies, coconut oil has shown promising results for treating diabetes and insulin resistance. As early as 1968, MCT (medium-chain triglycerides) found in coconut oil have been used in diabetic studies and reveal improvement in glucose tolerance.[26]

I am a purist when it comes to oils. I want to consume oils in their very purest state. I only use oils that are minimally processed. As stated in my first book, I don't condone the use of canola oil, mostly because it undergoes quite a bit of processing to become safe for consumption. Pure canola oil contains erucic acid, an omega-9 fatty acid that makes the oil bitter. Omega-9 fatty acids promote inflammation in the body.

Canola oil is processed at high temperatures to remove the erucic acid; therefore, the processing alone causes a risk of rancidity and oxidation. Cold-pressed oils such as cold-pressed olive oil and cold-pressed sesame oil are much better, healthier oils. If you're using cold-pressed sesame oil, add it to the food right before serving to avoid heating the oil too high. Use olive oil for light sautéing only. At moderate temperatures it does an okay job of withstanding heat. For cooking at higher temperatures or for a prolonged time, I use mostly coconut oil or, occasionally, a little organic butter. For most oils, if the label does not say cold-pressed, you can assume that heat and possibly chemicals were involved in the extraction process and you should stay away.

Grape seed oil is processed from the seeds of grapes, which are formed as a by-product of wine making. Oftentimes, oils like this are a great idea for businesses that want to make something out of their discarded product. Grape seed oil is a mostly polyunsaturated fat that isn't able to withstand high heat. Grape seed oil is high in omega-6 fatty acids. Now, we do need some omega-6 fatty acids in our diet, but the usual ratio of omega-3 fatty acid to omega-6 fatty acid is disproportionate in the American diet already; therefore, I do not push the consumption of omega-6 fatty acids.

Palm oil is still too controversial and not well enough understood for me to add it to my and my family's diet, especially because olive oil, coconut oil, and a little bit of organic butter provide all the oils we need.

Monounsaturated fats, which I mentioned earlier, have been the subject of a large amount of positive research touting their cardiac benefits. This is especially true of research conducted on the Mediterranean-type diet, which has shown the favorable effects of consuming large amounts of olive oil, a monounsaturated fat. Monounsaturated fats have very loose double bonds that keep the oil liquid at room temperature, unlike saturated fats, which are more solid at room temperature. Monounsaturated fats are easier for the body to break down and digest due to their double-bond struc-ture. For this reason, they are also very unstable during cooking. I suggest including monounsaturated fats in your diet but heating them in only rare instances. It is best to start sautéing and cooking with water and using olive oil in your salad dressings or to drizzle over a meal before serving. Olive oil is also great in dips and sprinkled over vegetables.

Eggs

Eggs and their nutrition content versus their potential harm have been a subject of confusion for decades. Many people worry that eggs are high in cholesterol; therefore, they avoid them if they have cholesterol problems. Eating eggs in moderation can be a great source of protein. Eggs contain saturated fat, but we do need some saturated fats in our diet, and eggs are a better choice than other types of saturated fats. Eggs are also high in lecithin, which is protective for fat metabolism. One egg can have as much as 2,000 mg of lecithin. Lecithin's ability to shuttle fats into and out of cells has been shown to promote healthy cholesterol levels. It emulsifies cholesterol (makes it mix with other fluids in the body, such as blood) before it can attach to cell walls and start clogging arteries. Strangely enough, the same emulsifying properties that make lecithin important in condiments may make it helpful in preventing strokes, heart attacks, and arteriosclerosis. Lecithin acts like motor oil for your nervous system, keeping everything lubricated and firing away smoothly and efficiently, which translates into faster reaction times and improved body function. As an added bonus, it may even help you metabolize fat.

Consuming organic, hormone-free eggs is okay! I eat eggs often, and my HDL cholesterol is over 100 and my LDL is under 100. Many of my patients with perfect cholesterol numbers have followed the anti-inflammatory diet, which includes eggs, for nearly a decade.

In recent years, a number of studies have supported the healthfulness of egg consumption. For example, a recent study conducted in Finland found that egg consumption was associated with lower risk for type 2 diabetes and improved blood glucose control. The study, published in the *Journal of Clinical Nutrition,* revealed that men who ate four or more eggs per week had a 37 percent lower risk than men who only ate one egg per week. Thirty-seven percent is a significant margin, and I will take my chances and enjoy my eggs.[27]

Essential Fatty Acids

Essential fatty acids, EFAs, are necessary fats that the human body cannot synthesize; they must be obtained through foods or supplements. EFAs are long-chain polyunsaturated fatty acids derived from linolenic, linoleic, and oleic acids. Polyunsaturated fats are even more fluid than monounsaturated fats because they are composed of many loose double bonds. There are two families of EFAs: omega-3 and omega-6. (Omega-9 fatty acids are necessary but are not considered "essential" because the body can synthesize them if they are not obtained through diet.)

Omega-6 fats, found in a variety of nuts and seeds, are common in our diets. Omega-3 fats occur less commonly. In most diets nowadays, omega-3 fats need to be sought out. They are, in my opinion, the superior type of EFA because of their direct anti-inflammatory properties. Omega-6 fats feed the inflammatory pathway in most individuals but play an important role in immune system balance as well. Therefore, omega-6 fats are vital, but because they are already abundant and even in excess in the diet, consuming more omega-6 fats may, in fact, trigger the inflammatory cascade.

EFAs are studied regularly in regard to cardiac health; a recent study demonstrated their ability to reduce the risk of stroke and heart attack. Additionally, the ratio of omega-6 to omega-3 fatty acids has recently been studied in regard to cardiovascular health. The study, published in *Experimental Biology and Medicine*, reports that a lower ratio of omega-6 fatty acids to omega-3 fatty acids is favorable for reducing cardiovascular disease as well as other chronic diseases. This study pointed out that a higher intake of omega-3 fatty acids, compared with omega-6 fatty acids, was favorable. Even with the same amount of omega-3 intake, if omega-6 fatty acids were increased, the protective effect of omega-3 fatty acids was negated.[28] This brings up an important point. We are so supplement hungry in our society. Oftentimes, people think taking their omega-3 fatty acids daily is protective, but they haven't considered what they are putting into their bodies. This supports once again that changing your risk does not mean changing only one habit or making only one dietary change, but involves a combination of many lifestyle changes. Putting the time in to live a complete program can be much more beneficial than just supporting one leg of the proverbial three-legged stool. Things will still remain pretty "tippy" if you only do a couple of improvements—like taking a supplement—without the others—exercise and dietary management.

Our Environment Is No Longer Clean

The long list of irritants that may trigger a chronic inflammatory response includes substances that were never meant to be ingested or absorbed by our bodies. We have created a toxic environment that can cause illness after long-term exposure, especially if those effects are not counteracted with positive lifestyle measures. Just a few of the offending substances are:

- air pollutants
- alcohol
- chemicals added to cosmetics, lotions, and other body-care products
- chemicals in unfiltered water
- food additives/food dyes (e.g., MSG)
- harsh cleaning chemicals
- heavy metals such as mercury, lead, and fluoride
- hormones, such as the synthetic chemicals added to animal feed to encourage growth
- nicotine and chemicals added to cigarettes
- over-the-counter medications
- pesticides and herbicides
- pharmaceutical/prescription drugs
- preservatives of all kinds (contained in many products, from skin products to food to lawn products and many others)
- radon
- street drugs
- xenoestrogen chemicals and other endocrine disrupters such as bisphenol-A (BPA)

All these dangerous substances, and many more that aren't listed here, pose a potential threat to the body. When exposed to such toxins, the body responds naturally by attacking. The attack may be so small in scale that you can't feel it or sense it. Often, the response may fail to show up on a blood test until a person is well into an illness but this may truly be the beginning of chronic inflammatory responses in the body.

When I think about the amount of toxicity we have been exposed to since conception, I consider how clouded our receptor sites are for signaling molecules, neurotransmitters, and hormones in the body. The more toxic the body is, the more clouded those receptors become. When toxicity in the body is constant, isn't removed, or is in excess, the receptors begin to malfunction and don't do as good a job of accepting their signaling molecule. This is extremely important in basic metabolism of all body processes, and if these processes are inhibited or depressed, then you might feel suboptimal. Suboptimal functioning of the body will lead to suboptimal physiology and health in all aspects, mentally, emotionally, and physically. You remember the saying "moving through molasses"? This is how I picture the body when it is under toxin stress. Optimizing the body to eliminate toxicity properly, in addition to avoiding excess toxins in food, pharmaceutical medications, and the environment, can improve body functions and health.

One example of how toxicity affects receptor function is the use of quinolones. Quinolones are a family of compounds used as broad-spectrum antibiotics. In a research study published in the *Journal of Antimicrobial Chemotherapy* in 1990, the use of quinolones were found to have convulsion-like effects on mice, and the suspected mechanism was the displacement of GABA from its receptor sites.[29] GABA is an extremely important molecule in preventing anxiety and promoting relaxation and sleep. I could find hundreds of more studies to support the problem with receptor function and interfering compounds. What you need to understand is that the more junk you put into your body, the more chance you have of interfering with important physiological processes needed for optimal health.

Because I believe hormones are extremely important to vitality, slowing down the effects of aging, improved quality of life, and decreased risk for future chronic illnesses, it is extremely important that we keep the receptors for all hormones clean and functioning well. Another good example of receptor problems arising in the body is insulin resistance. Excess sugar in the bloodstream can cause issues with the receptors on cells for insulin and result in the body needing to use more insulin and consequently requiring more receptors to do the same job insulin was supposed to be doing at lower concentrations and with fewer receptors. Insulin resistance will be discussed in detail in future chapters.

Quality of Grown Food

The quality of our food supply is fast deteriorating. Due to deficient soil quality, as well as the number of chemicals used on and around plants, the health of the food we grow and produce has suffered. Pesticides, herbicides, and other fertilizers have caused our vegetables to undergo changes that make the food less digestible. Genetically engineering food to be "tougher" in the environment, such as against weather conditions, molds, or insects, makes the food tougher to digest. Genetic engineering is also used to make vegetables bigger, to allow them to grow outside their normal temperature zones, etc. When genetic engineering changes the food, it also changes how we digest the food. As the food gets more and more foreign to what we are used to, it becomes less digestible. Let's not forget the lack of nutrients caused by altering the gene structure of the food.

Foods are now shipped large distances and lose the vitality they had when they were just picked. Food is sprayed, irradiated, and processed for easy consumption and to improve market share for mass-producing farmers and companies. Meat quality has also changed drastically. From the very early meat of hunters and gatherers, the meat has taken on a significantly higher fat content due to our grain-intensive feeding procedures. During hunter-and-gatherer days, the meat that was hunted was only fatty during particular seasons when the animals were ready to go into hibernation. Most other times of the year, animal meats were made of lean muscle mass. Additionally, animal proteins have become heavily processed. The feed used is not only grain, but grain treated with antibiotics and sometimes growth hormones, producing significantly larger animals than nature intended. All this additional bulking-up of animals is targeted at producing the highest amount of profit. After all, raising animals for consumption is now a large business, and businesses want to be profitable.

In my past, I worked for an agriculture company that worked with chicken and pig farms. We were trying to develop probiotic washes that could be used on the bedding in poultry houses to keep them from getting breast blisters. It was very interesting work and I thought we were contributing to a better good from our end. It wasn't until my first time in the chicken house that my eyes were opened to why in the world their bedding needed to be treated. The chickens were overfed until they were rather large, and some couldn't stand up anymore, so they ended up resting on their bedding. Obviously, if their bedding was treated with a better probiotic blend, it would help reduce the blisters that they acquired on their breast tissue, the part of their body that lay on the bedding. I bring this point up because we are mass-producing everything we can in order to make profit. It is almost like survival of the fittest has really set in. Who can survive the low-quality food and sedentary lifestyle that America and other nations have adopted? Who can survive the leaking of nuclear radiation from the Fukushima fallout in Japan? Who can buy up the most stocks to ensure they have an edge over other nations? Who can produce the most profit by spending the least amount of money? It isn't about food quality anymore; it is about mass production and convenience. Many people are busy, and convenience foods are easy, quick, and relatively inexpensive. Organic food costs more and is sometimes hard to find. Due to the deficient nutrient quality of the soil, even organic food may still lack the nutrients that foods once had. I am not going to lie: making healthy food takes a little time, but the longer you do it, the better you get at it and the better you get at making a healthy meal in a pinch. I often say to my patients that they should have some go-to meals that they can make when they have to work fast. These meals should be relatively quick to prepare, healthy, and taste good; otherwise they won't be your go-to meals for long.

We Can't Meet All Our Needs with Supplements

Because soil is deficient and foods are laden with chemicals, should we just take a lot of supplements to ward off deficiencies? This is certainly not what I am saying, but I am saying that we have to work a lot harder at getting nutrients out of our diet in this day and age compared to years ago. Additionally, due to the excessive chemicals in our environment and food, our bodies have to do quite a bit of work just processing and eliminating the unwanted material. Supplements can be great and are important additions to treatment plans, but they do not take the place of healthy diet and lifestyle. In addition, many supplements are not the quality you may think they are. For example, many supplements don't actually contain the amount of herb or vitamin listed on the label. There are not a lot of regulations for supplements in the United States, so supplements can be poor quality.

Additionally, many supplements contain additional material unlisted on the label. Herbs that are imported often are not purified and can contain heavy metals and other chemicals. If the supplement company using these bulk materials does not check the quality of the ingredients they are using, then the unwanted material gets manufactured right into the product (often without the maker of the supplement knowing that their product is contaminated). It is extremely important to know the quality of the supplements that you are taking in. Make sure you can trust the company you are buying from. You can even go a step further and discuss with the company their testing methods for both their bulk material and their finished product. If they are willing to discuss it or send you a quality-control assay, I would say they are a pretty good company.

Sometimes, we go supplement crazy and take too many at a time. Our body cannot digest that many at once. I don't tolerate my patients taking something like 12 supplements at a time because it just creates work for the body. When you take that many supplements, it is hard for your body to metabolize them, just as it is hard for the body to metabolize multiple medications. Any time you add a substance to the body, even if it is a supplement, the body has to work to process it. Some supplements or hormone replacements are necessary for patients; I am just cautioning you against the use of a broad-spectrum, "hit-your-body-with-everything" approach to supplementing. I feel it can do the body harm in the long run. Additionally, when you use supplements with more directed actions and don't start them all at the same time, you are better able to assess your improvement on the supplement or few you are taking.

Choosing the Right Number of Supplements

Due to our stark nutrient deficiencies, I do believe that some amount of supplementation is needed to accelerate the movement toward better health. Antioxidants are important for maintaining healthy internal functioning, supporting proper brain neurochemicals, and keeping the arteries and other tissues safe from free-radical damage. Probiotics are not readily available in the standard diets unless someone is regularly consuming kimchi, raw sauerkraut, kefir, kombucha, or other fermented foods. Essential fatty acids are so low in the diet that they often need to be supplemented to get enough anti-inflammatory benefit in inflammation-related conditions (which you have already learned are most conditions). A healthy body may not require as much supplement support, but a body that is already in a diseased state may require supplementation in addition to a healthy diet and lifestyle program to facilitate a quicker response to therapies. In Chapter 12, I outline an effective supplement plan to implement with the diet change. You can either take the supplements along with the diet and lifestyle changes or you can make the diet and exercise changes only. The diet alone will make significant blood sugar changes if you stick to it consistently. It will take longer for the blood sugar to normalize without the supplement program, but it can occur. I suggest that if you are not planning on taking the supplements, you follow the diet for a longer period of time before introducing foods back into the diet, and make sure that exercise is a vital part of your lifestyle commitment.

The Importance of Children's Health on Their Future

When a body is no longer in homeostasis for any reason—improper diet, poor lifestyle habits, genetic family history, chronic emotional stress, environmental toxin overload, or sedentary life-style—it becomes weaker, rendering it less able to defend itself against certain microorganisms and other disease states such as inflammation, aging, and diabetes. We call this general state of bodily reactivity and health one's "terrain." Based on the strength of one's terrain, disease can be either avoided or inevitable.

If we have a strong belief in maintaining a healthy terrain, it follows that we want to promote health in our children. As children grow bigger and stronger, the insides of their bodies are also developing in important ways that we are unable to see. A child's nervous system, brain, and immune system develop throughout childhood. To promote optimal health and development, it is important to protect children's terrains through proper diet and lifestyle. If we focus on minimizing pesticide residues, hormones, and antibiotic residues in foods; including nutritive foods as part of a balanced diet; eliminating food allergies; and eliminating sugars, white flour, and other immune-suppressive foods, children will be much healthier in the long run.

Consider this: from 1980 to 2011, the number of people in the United States diagnosed with diabetes more than tripled. According to the 2014 National Diabetes Statistics Report put out by the Centers for Disease Control and Prevention, 29 million people in the United States have diabetes. This accounts for 9.3 percent of our population! I will tell you right now, this imbalance in sugar metabolism begins early, as early as childhood. Children consuming sugary foods and drinking soda or juice have a significant risk of becoming insulin resistant and are more likely to develop diabetes in the future. Knowing what to keep our children away from in their developmental years is vital to their future health.

If we promote a healthy lifestyle from the start, many children will remain disease free. I believe it is my responsibility to my child to keep her healthy in order to prevent future chronic disease. It is also important to offer children a loving, supportive atmosphere in which to grow and develop, because as you will learn in chapters to come, emotions play an important role in health and disease.

There is one more thing to note about a child's development. When a child is faced with a bacterial or viral insult and gets a cold, flu, or fever, it is a positive reaction. It allows us to see that the child's body is able to react against foreign antigens. It is important for children to get sick and to mount fevers a few times per year. As this happens, the immune system is "practicing" and developing. In our medical practice we often observe that after a child has gone through an illness, he or she will do something new. He or she may say a new word, take his or her first step, learn a new skill, act with a little more conviction about things, or build more self-confidence. This is a truly amazing aspect of childhood development; children develop as their immune response develops. If we damp down the immune response with Tylenol, antibiotics, or any other suppressive treatment, we are telling the body not to react and thus not to practice developing its immune response. If we suppress children's reactions enough times, the body will stop reacting.

The immune system has many components, and if all components are not exercised and developed, the system can become out of balance. The child whose immune response has been suppressed too often may stop having minor infection reactions such as colds and flus. Suppressing the proper reaction of the immune system in children allows them to be exposed to many foreign invaders that are never fended off. If these invaders are stored instead of eliminated from the body, they have the potential to cause future health problems.

Bottom line: Any imbalance in immune function, such as prolonged exposure to foreign invaders without ridding the body of them, can increase chronic inflammation, decrease the ability to fight off foreign invaders, and increase the potential for autoimmune reactions, elevations in inflammation, and chronic disease.

CHAPTER 2

Gastrointestinal Health Is Essential to Survival

The gastrointestinal tract is where nutrient exchange occurs and where our body takes in what it needs from the outside world. Granted, the lungs do this also, taking in oxygen, but the GI tract is where the health of the body begins. The GI tract is part of a significant number of intricate and vital mechanisms that create a whole host of reactions and interactions. The GI lining, being as thin as your eyelid, is one of the busiest organs of your body. Always concerned with transport, it must do the difficult job of greeting all new chemicals that enter your mouth via food and drink to initiate digestion and absorption of the needed nutrients, and rejection of foreign material the body does not want to allow into the bloodstream.

The lining of the GI tract is also the central hub of the immune system. As mentioned above, it is where the decisions are made in determining "who" is friend and foe, the chemicals that we should let in and gain nutrients from and the chemicals we should mount a reaction against. This is called building oral tolerance. This is an important process of the immune system that determines our reactions towards certain foods, chemicals, bacteria, viruses, and so forth. The body should naturally begin to understand what to react to and what not to react to starting with chemicals through breast milk and then from food introduction on. When the GI lining is confused, it may become hypervigilant in its attack against many compounds, sometimes promoting attack against chemicals that don't cause the body harm. Usually this is when we see multiple food allergies, auto-immune conditions, and other allergies in patients. The GI tract has lost its ability to know whom to let in and whom to keep out, including sometimes its own cells, as in autoimmune conditions. When the health of the gastrointestinal tract improves, allergies lessen, digestion improves, and immune recognition improves.

Probiotics in the Gastrointestinal Tract

The process of understanding what items to allow in and what items to reject can be difficult for the body, especially if probiotic balance is off. Probiotics are important bacteria, yeasts, and micro-organisms that line our gastrointestinal tract. In fact, you have many more microorganisms lining your gastrointestinal tract than the body has cells. Your microflora (the balance of your gastrointestinal microorganisms) is extremely important for digestion. First of all, the microorganisms are the first line of defense that your food encounters, and they predigest our food. By creating a wonderfully efficient symbiotic relationship, we allow our microflora to stay and flourish within our gastrointestinal systems. If the important job of predigesting foods is done well, then the food particles that are presented to the GI lining are small and manageable and can easily be further broken down into nutrients, which are then allowed to cross the gastrointestinal tract.

When probiotic balance is disrupted—for example, after anti-biotics or from repeated courses of antibiotics—this important predigestion can be inhibited or diminished. If this occurs, then larger food particles are presented to the GI lining and, after repeated offenses, can affect the strength of the GI lining. The GI lining is dependent on gap junctions between each cell in the lining main-taining very tight control of the border into the bloodstream. Various insults can affect these gap junctions and the tight border control, such as large food particles, anti-inflammatory medications (think NSAIDs), and other pharmaceutical medications, as well as a host of other offending chemicals. For instance, gluten is a well-known catalyst of increased intestinal permeability, which is why the Freedom Diet is so important to injured GI tracts.

The GI Tract Is Our First Immune System

Not only is the gastrointestinal lining our barrier from the outside world; it also has, its very own immune system. The GALT, gut-associated lymphatic tissue, is truly its own high-functioning immune system with the sole job of protecting the body from invasion. For example, if a harmful bacterium or virus comes into the GI tract, the GALT is the system responsible for mounting the important immune system attack on the foreign invader. The GALT system can be subject to confusion when autoimmune diseases are present.

The GI Tract's Role in Emotional Health

The gastrointestinal tract is the hub for many neurotransmitters. For example, one neurotransmitter extremely important in mood, serotonin, is found largely in the gut. In fact, 90–95 percent of the body's serotonin is located in the gut. Serotonin in the gut inhibits acid secretion and promotes gastric and intestinal mucus production. Serotonin may affect gastrointestinal blood flow and can play a role in the pathogenesis of diarrhea and other GI disorders. What this brings to mind is how connected your GI tract is to your mood and emotional health. Serotonin in the gut may, in fact, have an effect on how much serotonin is in circulation and able to affect the central nervous system and neurons throughout the body. Interestingly, we can think of our gut as our "second brain." This little brain in your abdomen can have a significant amount to do during the day. The nerve network in the GI tract can have as many as 100 million neurons, more than in either the spinal cord or the peripheral nervous system. Although you won't be generating any thoughts in the GI tract, you can certainly feel your emotions at work in your gut sometimes. You get a little nervous or excited about something and feel it in your gut, right? Another interesting connection is that many of the nerves in the gut are nerves that send messages to the brain, but there are not a lot of nerves coming from the brain to the gut. This makes us assume that the gut has its own defined nervous system for performing its daily tasks without having to get continual input from the brain. We may consider then that our everyday emotional state is reliant on messages from the gut to the brain. It isn't by chance that many medications targeted at improving the mood, such as SSRIs (selective serotonin reuptake inhibitors), also come with gastrointestinal side effects.

Think of the gastrointestinal tract's relationship to the emotions as a barrier. The GI lining is responsible for figuring out who is friend and who is foe and working hard to maintain the barrier and maintain the body's health and integrity. The GI lining needs to understand what bacteria and food are beneficial and what viruses, foreign material, and parasites are harmful. Likewise, we have to focus on our emotional balance daily, figuring out which situations and people cause us to feel emotionally healthy and which situations and people we should avoid.

Most people process their emotions in a manner similar to how their gastrointestinal tract processes its food and maintains its functions. If someone is regularly constipated, they will often be emotional stuffers as well, meaning they hold their emotions in. Additionally, when someone is constipated they often will have symptoms like migraines or anxiety. If someone doesn't have a problem with their bowel movements, they may not be as likely to stuff their emotions. If someone is plagued with regular anxiety, they may experience times of diarrhea. We can understand this by looking at children. When they get nervous, where do they feel it? Most of the time, they will have a upset stomach. These are just a few examples of many in which the gastrointestinal tract is intimately connected to our emotional health and vice versa.

Time and time again, by improving the health of the gastrointestinal tract and improving its ability to maintain its barrier, we improve our emotions. If we can promote better boundaries within a person's GI tract, his or her emotional boundaries get better as well. As the GI lining is healthier, hormones are secreted more efficiently and emotions can stay better controlled.

CHAPTER 3

Inflammation's Impact on Health

Predominant Illnesses in Our Society and throughout the World

You know someone who has had a heart attack, you know someone who's lost a loved one to cardiac disease, you know someone who has diabetes or you yourself have it, and you have encountered someone with cancer. These diseases are rampant throughout our society, and a large cause of them is our habits. We spend so much time worrying about how to fight off bacterial infections, the common cold, flus, and other minor illnesses, but do we stop to think about the health of our internal environment? Most of my patients are only worried about the day-to-day things. People tend to think about their sleep, energy, the cold they need to ward off because they have to get to work, and making sure they can continue their strenuous schedules. They are not concerned with their impending future illnesses. Because of this lack of concern in our general society, I haven't seen great strides taken by many people to change their diets or lifestyle habits. Now this is not true of everyone. Many of my patients are exercising daily and eating healthily, and they are very concerned about making sure they have good future health. I am even starting to do risk panels on my patients so we can better understand their cardiovascular risks. I am doing this in people as early as their teens and 20s so that we can do a better job of preventing future imbalances.

Take heart disease, for example. It is still the number-one cause of death by illness in the United States and, in fact, is the most fatal illness in the world. Heart disease is often a silent illness. Many times there are no symptoms at all. If someone isn't doing regular blood panels and isn't visiting a physician, then minor changes in blood pressure and/or blood tests won't be observed, and nothing can be done to help improve cardiovascular health and decrease risk for illness. Especially in women, the first symptom of heart disease can be death. So I am here to say now that it is more important than ever to change diet and lifestyle habits.

As of 2013, according to the CDC, the top 10 leading causes of death in the United States are:

- heart disease: 611,105
- cancer: 584,881
- chronic lower respiratory diseases: 149,205
- accidents (unintentional injuries): 130,557
- stroke (cerebrovascular diseases): 128,978
- Alzheimer's disease: 84,767
- diabetes: 75,578
- influenza and pneumonia: 56,979
- nephritis, nephrotic syndrome, and nephrosis: 47,112
- intentional self-harm (suicide): 41,149[30]

Almost all of these are directly related to inflammation. The only two causes of death I can spare from inflammatory causes are accidents and intentional self-harm, and I can connect both indirectly to increased levels of oxidative stress and inflammation. Indirectly, inflammation and accidents are related because many of the accidents in this category occur in hospitals or involve pharmaceutical prescription errors. My guess is that many of the medications with which doctors make prescribing errors or patients make consumption errors are for conditions with inflammation at the root. Additionally, many patients are in the hospital tending to illnesses that are directly related to inflammation when some of these accidents occur. On another note, accidents also involve auto accidents, some of which occur due to the health problems of an individual causing them to pass out. When I wrote my second book, *More Anti-Inflammation Diet Tips and Recipes*, I was shocked to see that the tenth leading health threat was suicide/attempted suicide. These 2013 statistics match the 2009 statistics listed in that book, with intentional self-harm still registering as one of the top 10. Current research suggests that lifestyle factors that affect inflammation also can affect one's sense of well-being. Extreme oxidative stress has an impact on the balance of neurochemicals that are needed for proper mood and stability. Neurotransmitters can be affected by the excess amount of oxidative stress that we experience through environmental insults, which can result in significant anxiety and depression. These mood imbalances can lead to increased risk for suicidal thoughts. It's important to address your mental and emotional well-being as part of a holistic approach to health. Suicide is often preceded by depression, anxiety, or bipolar tendencies. If you feel your emotions are out of control, please seek help to obtain the balance you need.

We all have a high likelihood of developing one of these health problems, each of which can lead to death. Of course, death is inevitable, but it's how we live until that moment that is important to me. We needn't live our lives resigned to the prospect of growing sicker and more disabled as we age. In a perfect world, one would be at one's healthiest for the longest time possible, then become ill and quickly perish without much suffering. It is my hope that individuals who care for themselves and their bodies attain this goal. It is not too late to take accountability for your habits and change them to enhance your future. You can also inspire your friends and associates to adopt healthier lifestyles by setting an example, and you can certainly influence your children's lifelong habits by introducing good practices into your home starting today.

Top 10 Leading Causes of Death in the World

Worldwide, we see many of the same illnesses plaguing most people, with the top four causes of death being ischemic heart disease, stroke, chronic obstructive pulmonary disease, and lower respiratory infections. Throughout the world, including the United States, diabetes is steadily increasing and heart disease stays the number-one killer. According to the World Health Organization, if you add up all-cause cardiac mortality, three out of every ten deaths in the world are cardiovascular in nature. In 2012, cardiovascular disease killed 17.5 million people worldwide! In the past decade, stroke and heart disease have continued to increase, but we have made some strides in reducing the number of deaths from lower respiratory tract infections, diarrheal illnesses, preterm birth complications, tuberculosis, and HIV/AIDs.

The top 10 leading causes of death in the world according to the WHO are:

- ischemic heart disease: 7.4 million
- stroke: 6.7 million
- chronic obstructive pulmonary diseases: 3.1 million
- chronic lower respiratory diseases: 3.1 million
- lung cancers, including cancers in the trachea and bronchus: 1.6 million
- HIV/AIDS: 1.5 million
- diarrheal illnesses: 1.5 million
- diabetes: 1.5 million
- road injury: 1.3 million
- hypertensive events: 1.1 million[31]

It is interesting to look at the leading causes of death in the world versus the United States. The United States is one of the most industrialized countries of the world. With this understanding, one can assume that the United States, with it's state-of-the-art acute treatment facilities and easy access the health care, succeeds at eliminating the numbers of deaths from infectious diseases such as tuberculosis, diarrhea, HIV/AIDs, and respiratory tract infections. Many of these infectious diseases may result in death more quickly in a third world nation with limited health care. Interestingly, though, as we see decreases in acute/infectious illnesses, or what I call "hot" diseases, we see "cold" diseases increase. I consider "cold" diseases to be the chronic illnesses of our time: cancer, heart disease, autoimmune disease, diabetes, stroke, arthritis, Alzheimer's disease, and other chronic illnesses.

Health Care across the Globe

The United States spends more on health care than any other country in the world. Numerous comparisons have been conducted between the United States and other countries to determine the effectiveness of our expansive and expensive health care system. According to the Commonwealth Fund's report *Mirror, Mirror on the Wall: How the Performance of the U.S. Healthcare System Compares Internationally*, for 2014, the United States consistently underperforms relative to other countries in most dimensions. The United States came in last in this recent comparison of eleven different nations, even though we spend the most. The other nations studied for the report were Australia, Canada, France, Germany, the Netherlands, New Zealand, Norway, Sweden, Switzerland, and the United Kingdom.[32] Previous editions of *Mirror, Mirror* from 2004, 2006, 2007, and 2010 reached the same conclusion: the United States is last or near last on dimensions of access, efficiency, and equity. The *Mirror, Mirror* report includes information from the three most recent Commonwealth Fund international surveys of patients and primary care physicians about medical practices and views of their country's health systems (2011–2013). It also includes information on health care outcomes featured in the Commonwealth Fund's most recent (2011) national health system scorecard, and from the WHO and the Organization for Economic Cooperation and Development.

Additionally, the current US vaccination schedule proposes 26 vaccine doses to be given to an infant before they turn one. This is more than any other country in the world! Yet 33 other nations are ranked ahead of us in infant mortality rates! Infant mortality rates are based on the amount of deaths that occur within the first year of a baby's life. That means we have more babies die in the first year of life compared to 33 other nations. And we spend the most on health care compared with anyone else in the world. Are we doing something wrong? Are all our interventions necessary, or are they causing more harm than good? I don't know the answer to these questions, but I do know that we need to understand that health care in the United States is not ideal and often is not correct. Therefore, continuing to heavily medicate without making drastic lifestyle and diet changes will send people to their graves, most likely with heart disease or cancer.

Inflammation's Influence on Illness and Health

Researchers are finding more and more evidence linking chronic inflammation with chronic disease. According to an article published in *Alternative Therapies in Health and Medicine,* cardiovascular disease, metabolic syndrome, hypertension, diabetes, and elevated cholesterol can be reversed by reversing the cause: inflammation caused by visceral fat tissue.[33] Alzheimer's disease has been connected to elevations in heavy metals. But since everyone living in a similar area is exposed to the same types of heavy metals throughout their lifetime, why are some individuals getting Alzheimer's and some not? This is mainly due to genetics, diet, lifestyle, and how well their bodies eliminate the heavy metals. Some people's bodies are better than others' at eliminating the oxidative stressors of daily life. Healthy habits will improve your body's ability to reduce the free-radical damage that can occur from everyday habits, stress, and environmental exposure.

Even healthy cells sometimes mount an immune response against normal cells, resulting in an inflammatory attack on certain tissues such as those found in joints, nerves, and connective tissue. This is how inflammation may be related to autoimmune conditions such as rheumatoid arthritis, multiple sclerosis, lupus, or psoriasis. Current research has helped us to understand that chronic inflammation is related to a host of illnesses, including some of the most deadly conditions worldwide. In this chapter, I want to help you understand inflammation. Why does it matter? How do we know that chronic inflammation is harmful? What is the difference between "good" and "bad" inflammation?

Inflammation plays an important role in our health. It is part of the intricate immune system, our body's first line of defense against bacteria, viruses, and other foreign invaders. Too much of a good thing, though, can be counterproductive and in some cases may prove deadly. Although the job of the immune system is to protect the body, when faced with long-term exposure to modern irritants like smoking, lack of exercise, and a diet of high-sugar, high-calorie, and highly processed foods, the inflammation process goes into overdrive. These are the circumstances under which inflammation causes harm to bodily tissues.

Inflammation at the Cellular Level
The Process of Inflammation

Inflammation is the first response by the immune system to infection or irritation. It presents with the cardinal signs of redness (Latin: *rubor*), heat (*calor*), swelling (*tumor*), pain (*dolor*), and dysfunction of the organs involved. Acute inflammation is needed to help heal acute trauma, abrasions, broken bones, or acute invasion of a foreign substance, such as bee venom from a bee sting. The body reacts immediately to acute trauma by increasing substances that stimulate swelling, redness, pain, and heat. These responses are important because they keep the body from doing further damage to the injury or wound by promoting pain and swelling all around the injured area. This causes an individual to be more cautious when moving the affected part.

For example, if you break your wrist, the pain and inflammation will force you to protect the wrist from the further damage that could occur if you used it or moved it too quickly. Sometimes acute inflammation can be triggered deeper in the body, for example when repairing a blood vessel. But if the lifestyle habits and environmental stressors that initiated the blood vessel damage in the first place are not changed, then the inflammation may remain present for a longer period of time. Consequently, we can see minor inflammation processes like this occurring in various places throughout the body, not just in blood vessels. The more places where you have low-grade inflammation, the worse off your prognosis will be going forward. Low-grade inflammation can be present in many tissues such as joints, muscles, the liver, blood vessels, skin, and others.

Chronic inflammation is an ongoing, low level of inflammation invisible to the human eye that usually occurs as a response to prolonged acute inflammation or repetitive injuries. Chronic inflammation is the underlying cause associated with most of the common causes of death in industrialized nations. It is unknown how inflammation begins in chronic disease, but there are many theories, some of which are discussed in this chapter.

Chronic inflammation can and will lead to necrosis (tissue destruction) by the inflammatory cells and by certain other agents. The body's healing response depends upon many factors, including persistent infection; the presence of foreign material or other agents that stimulate inflammation (such as latent viruses, bacteria, or parasites); lifestyle factors including diet, exercise, and sleep; inadequate blood supply; irradiation; and locally applied drugs such as corticosteroids. Other systemic factors include age (the healing process becomes slower and less effective with increasing age); deficiencies in nutrients such as vitamin C, zinc, and protein; chronic food allergies; metabolic diseases such as renal failure or diabetes mellitus; degenerative states associated with malignancies; and systemic drugs such as corticosteroids (these drugs can be used both topically and systemically).

A number of cells are important in the inflammatory cascade. The process of inflammation begins when the immune system triggers certain cells in the body to release cytokines, or proteins that send signals to other cells. Cytokines may be inflammation promoting or inflammation inhibiting. Cytokines that promote inflammation stimulate the release of immune cells locally (to one area of the body) or systemically (throughout the whole body).

The cells that release cytokines are known as leukocytes, or white blood cells; we generally think of them as our immune cells. In fact, there are several types of leukocytes, and all of them play a different role in the inflammatory process. It will be helpful to name just a few. Monocytes are cells that engulf foreign invaders or material. T lymphocytes, or T cells, help to initiate and direct the immune response and form memory responses for future infections. B lymphocytes help make antibodies needed for bacterial resistance. Lymphocytes are the cells that are often out of balance in inflammatory diseases.

These all-important leukocytes are produced and stored within the complex matrix of lymphatic tissue. The lymphatic system is comprised of the thymus gland, the spleen, the lymph nodes (located throughout the whole body), and the lymphatic tissue that lines the small intestine (called Peyer's patches, or aggregated lymphatic follicles). Lymphatic tissue and lymph nodes line every nerve and blood vessel in the body and function as a "highway" for immune cells and waste products. Immune cells use the lymphatic system to travel, repair, and fight. Wastes are constantly transported along the lymphatic system on their way to being exported through our main elimination organs: the kidneys, liver, gastrointestinal tract, and skin.

Making sure the lymphatic system is working properly is important in the treatment of all diseases because as we eliminate waste, it reduces stress on the elimination organs like the bowel, thereby supporting improved function. Accumulation of toxins in the bowel can confuse the immune response and promote autoimmune reactions or overreactions as well as suppressed immune responses.

Another important leukocyte is the mast cell. The cytokines released by mast cells recruit all the other types of immune cells to the site where the body is being attacked. The result is an immediate and robust inflammatory response. In the case of an injured ankle, for example, it is the mast cells that release the cytokines that cause the ankle to swell in as little as a minute after injury occurs. Mast cells appear to be the primary inflammatory mediator.

In addition to releasing cytokines, mast cells also secrete histamine, which is important in initiating local immune responses. Histamine is responsible for the irritation and redness you notice around a swollen bug bite. It stimulates blood vessels to allow larger quantities of white blood cells and proteins to pass through to an affected area. This helps facilitate a successful attack on foreign invaders or stimulate the healing response during an injury. We have come to understand, though, that histamine plays a much larger role in our general health and well-being.

Histamine

Histamine is good at stimulating the body to react, but it is sometimes responsible for heightening the response to an exaggerated or pathological degree. When histamine plays a part in a hyper-reaction, it is referred to as an allergic reaction. Allergic reactions can vary in severity from mild to lethal. Histamine is also a very stimulatory, or excitatory, molecule. It will heighten responses as well as heighten emotions such as anxiety. High histamine can be associated with depression as well. Medications known as antihistamines may reduce histamine and the allergic reactions caused by elevated histamine in the bloodstream, as well as promote sleep in many individuals. However, antihistamines have side effects, so if you find yourself using antihistamines daily for sleep or continued allergies, you should instead seek to reduce your need for them through diet changes, lifestyle changes, and a supplement routine so you can make a positive future health change. A recent study published in the *Journal of the American Medical Association* revealed the strongest evidence yet of the connection between increased risk for dementia and the use of anticholinergic drugs like Benadryl, NSAID nighttime medications like Tylenol PM, and over-the-counter allergy relief medications.[34] Interestingly, the study points out that these medications are being regularly used by at least 20 percent of our population.

Additionally, the risk is dose dependent, meaning the dosage and frequency with which the drug is used is related to a greater risk for dementia. The study further pointed out that even low doses, if used chronically, increase the risk for dementia. The study was conducted on older adults, the average age being 73 years, and their use was tracked backwards by 10 years. There hasn't been sufficient data on the use of these medications long-term in younger individuals. It is my understanding from my practice that many children are taking a daily allergy medication to control seasonal allergies and/or asthma. My suggestion for both adults and children is to find another way to cope with these issues and to reduce the use of anticholinergic drugs. Often if you remove all offending substances from the diet, the histamine reaction in the gut will decrease and overall allergy symptoms will diminish. They may improve dramatically or they may only lessen. Further treatment to balance the immune response may be necessary in some individuals to decrease their overall histamine response.

Histamine is an important neurotransmitter and can be a great marker to estimate methylation status. I discuss briefly the MTHFR gene and its effect on methylation in chapter 4. The MTHFR gene is currently being heavily studied by many physicians, who base their treatment plan for methyl status on it. Explained simply, methylation is the process of coding genes for proteins and enzymes that perform work in the body. The enzymes that promote a function's occurrence need to be properly stimulated in order for the function to occur optimally within the body. Many enzymes need a methyl group in order to continue with their function. When diets were healthier, prior to processing, methyl groups were obtained through diet and methylation reactions could occur more regularly.

Our genes play a huge part in how we methylate. The susceptibility to many mental, emotional, and psychiatric disorders can be directly linked to epigenetic inheritance. Some people are over-methylators and some are under-methylators.

Both of these methylation imbalances can be problematic to the consistent balance of neurotransmitters in the brain useful for balancing mood, sense of well-being, sleep, and energy. I describe it to my patients like this. Your enzymes are like the currency that you spend to make body processes happen optimally. If you are methylating properly, you take the 10-dollar bill out of your wallet and you spend it at the store and everything happens smoothly. You are even-keeled and in good spirits with the regular ups and downs because, for the most part, your brain neurochemistry is balanced. If you are over-methylating, it is like you have a clump of 10-dollar bills glued together in your wallet and when you want to spend them, you cannot because they're stuck together. This can result in an overabundance of brain neurotransmitters that can cause significant mental and emotional imbalance. Conversely, under-methylation occurs when you have the 10-dollar bill in your wallet but you can't get it out to spend it. You are deficient in important brain neurotransmitters that help to balance mood.

Eicosanoids and Inflammation

Inflammation, fever, tissue swelling, and allergies are largely controlled by fatty acids called eicosanoids. Eicosanoids are signaling molecules that have complex control over many bodily systems such as the growth and repair of tissues after offending events. These events could range from a signal sent during and after physical activity, inflammation or an immune response following the intake of toxic compounds and pathogens, or a message sent through the central nervous system. Eicosanoids are derived from either omega-6 or omega-3 fatty acids. The important eicosanoids we will discuss are prostaglandins and leukotrienes. There are three different families of prostaglandins that serve three different functions in the body. You can think of PGE_1 and PGE_3 as the "good" prostaglandins and PGE_2 as the proinflammatory or "bad" prostaglandin.

The following descriptions are presented for further understanding:

- PGE1 helps to reduce allergies, prevents inflammation, increases mucous production in the stomach, decreases blood pressure, improves nerve function, and helps to promote immune response.
- PGE2 stimulates the allergy response, promotes inflammation, increases platelet aggregation (when platelets stick to the site of plaque formations along blood vessel walls, leading to the development of localized blood clots, which can further block the flow of blood in the artery), increases smooth-muscle contraction, and suppresses immune function.
- PGE3 blocks the release of proinflammatory prostaglandins (PGE2), promotes immune function, decreases platelet aggregation, increases HDL cholesterol (the "good" cholesterol), decreases triglycerides, and inhibits inflammation.

There are two important leukotrienes that we will discuss: LBT4 and LBT5. You can think of LBT4 as the "bad" leukotriene and LBT5 as the "good" leukotriene:

- LBT4 is mainly a proinflammatory eicosanoid.
- LBT5 helps to decrease inflammation.

As you might expect, certain foods can promote production of prostaglandins and leukotrienes. Linoleic acid (from safflower oil, sunflower oil and seeds, sesame oil and seeds, and breast milk) can be converted into PGE_1, an anti-inflammatory pathway, or into arachidonic acid. Arachidonic acid (also from meats, dairy products, and breast milk) is converted into PGE_2 and LBT_4. Alpha-linolenic acid (from pumpkin seeds, flaxseeds, walnuts, soybeans, and breast milk) is converted into PGE_3 and LBT_5, thereby suppressing inflammation. Eicosapentaenoic acid (EPA) and docosahexaenoic acid (DHA) can be made by the body from alpha-linolenic acid (ALA). EPA and DHA promote the PGE_3 pathway (the "good" pathway) and are found in breast milk and cold-water fish such as salmon, mackerel, sardines, and trout.

Having an understanding of the inflammatory cascade and the way foods can influence inflammatory pathways in the body allows us to understand the importance of nutrient intake on how our body functions as a whole. Of special note is the fact that the enzymatic reaction that converts linoleic acid and alpha-linoleic acid into their metabolites is driven by the exact same enzyme, delta-6 desaturase. There is intense competition for this enzyme's use, especially because our diets are so linoleic heavy. Therefore, if we include plenty of alpha-linoleic-rich nuts and seeds, and DHA- and EPA-rich cold-water fish in our diets, we will naturally be inhibiting inflammation. Consuming these foods will increase PGE_3 and LBT_5 levels, which will in turn inhibit the formation of PGE_2 and LBT_4, the inflammatory prostaglandins.

The bodily enzymes involved in creating prostaglandins and arachidonic acid metabolites are of great importance with regard to the use of anti-inflammatory medication. For example, the important enzyme phospholipase A_2 (PLA_2) allows arachidonic acid to be released from cell membranes. Arachidonic acid production is the first step in promoting inflammation. Another enzyme, cyclooxygenase, is needed to convert arachidonic acid into PGE_2, prostacyclins, and thromboxanes, all of which promote inflammation. (Hint: You can tell a substance is an enzyme if its name ends in –*ase*.) Lipoxygenase is needed to promote the conversion of arachidonic acid into many other inflammation-producing prostaglandins. The cyclooxygenase-1 pathway helps in the formation of the stomach lining, and the cyclooxygenase-2 pathway promotes inflammation. Many anti-inflammation drugs affect both cyclooxygenase pathways, and thus harm the stomach lining. This topic is discussed in more detail later.

Inflammation and Chronic Diseases

Inflammation affects our health in more ways than one. We best understand its connection to heart disease but also understand that it has a direct influence on cancer, autoimmune diseases, arthritis, osteoporosis, and diabetes. In February of 2004, *Time* magazine featured a cover article on the connection between certain chronic diseases and inflammation. For example, evidence continues to show the clear connection between rheumatoid arthritis and other chronic inflammatory conditions and increased risk for heart disease. As you can guess, the increased inflammation present in rheumatoid patients puts them at increased risk of cardiac disease due to the damaging effect of the consistent inflammation on their vasculature and other important organs. Not only does inflammation cause damage in vascular organs and tissues; inflammation causes damage throughout all body tissues.[35] This information should not be new to us. In fact, I have found studies from as early as the 1960s discussing the connection between rheumatoid arthritis and heart health. This was even before we determined that the connection between these two conditions is, in fact, inflammation.[36]

The inflammation that started out so benign has now run rampant in our systems, wreaking havoc. I look at inflammation as I would a child who is allowed to run around the building without any discipline. They don't understand they are doing damage because no one is telling them to stop. When the inflammation in a person's body increases, there are no body processes telling the inflammation to stop. Overconsumption of inflammatory foods, toxic burden on the body, and damage within the body all continue to stimulate inflammatory processes.

Risk Factors for Increased Inflammation

Inflammation causes damage and can also cause confusion in the immune system. Initially, inflammation may not be causing damage that you can feel or see or be able to detect, but eventually inflammation is going to take its toll. Here are some symptoms and habits to look for that may indicate you are at risk of developing, or may already have, inflammation:

- chronic sinusitis
- chronic infections, especially if long-term and untreated
- arthritis of any type
- muscle or joint pain
- skin rashes, especially if present long-term
- hive-like rashes
- asthma
- diabetes, especially if poorly controlled
- family history of heart disease
- gum disease
- heart disease
- obesity or excessive weight
- poor diet
- sedentary lifestyle, lack of regular exercise
- smoking
- chronic high-stress lifestyle
- chronic diarrhea

The Harm in Chronic Use of Anti-Inflammatory Medications

When someone is in pain, it is common that the individual self-treat with or be prescribed anti-inflammatory medications such as steroid drugs or nonsteroidal anti-inflammatory drugs (also known as NSAIDs). Steroid-based anti-inflammatory drugs inhibit the immune system and interfere with the healing process. The NSAID group includes aspirin, ibuprofen (marketed under the names Motrin and Advil), and naproxen (Aleve). It does not include acetaminophen (Tylenol), which is effective against pain and fever but not against inflammation. Aspirin, ibuprofen, and naproxen inhibit the cyclo-oxygenase enzymes that promote the production of inflammatory mediators (mentioned above). However, because these drugs are not specific, they also affect the stomach lining, resulting in the possible side effects of ulcers and gastric (stomach) upset. In addition, NSAIDs block the release of the more anti-inflammatory prostaglandins, PGE_1 and PGE_3, which is contrary to the effect the drug is designed to produce.

Newer anti-inflammatory medications such as rofecoxib (Vioxx) mainly affect the cyclooxygenase-2 pathway; accordingly, they are called COX-2 inhibitors. These drugs are designed to spare the cyclooxygenase pathway that promotes stomach-lining health. They help with gastrointestinal side effects, but they have not reduced them completely and are not without their own side effects. And they still promote the lipoxygenase pathway of inflammatory-promoting substances. In September 2004, the Food and Drug Administration recalled Vioxx due to its causing an increased risk of cardiovascular events, including heart attack and stroke. Since then, Celebrex, also a COX-2 inhibitor and Vioxx's major competitor, has also raised eyebrows. Its manufacturer, Pfizer, has revealed that it halted a study in December of 2004 linking Celebrex to a "statistically significant" increase in cardiovascular risk. This was at least the second study that showed increased heart problems with the use of Celebrex.

A study published in the *British Medical Journal* in 2005 suggested that regular ingestion of rofecoxib, diclofenac, and ibuprofen significantly increased the risk of having a heart attack. No evidence was found proving that naproxen caused any increased risk for cardiovascular problems. This study and many others in the medical literature offer enough evidence to raise concerns about the cardiovascular safety of all NSAID use.

NSAIDs also have noncardiac side effects such as swelling, rashes, asthma, angioedema (deep swelling beneath the skin), urticaria (hives), anaphylaxis (a potentially life-threatening type of allergic reaction), and many more. It makes sense to adopt a healthy diet that will naturally decrease inflammation rather than relying on the long-term use of anti-inflammatory medications.

CHAPTER 4

The Importance of Blood Sugar

Insulin Resistance and Metabolic Syndrome

Insulin is a hormone secreted by the pancreas. The pancreas is an organ that sits behind your stomach on the left side of your abdominal cavity. Insulin is secreted by beta islet cells, and its main function is to control metabolism. We can think of metabolism as the way the body utilizes energy from food for body processes. When carbohydrates such as starches and sugars are consumed, they are broken down into glucose, the form of sugar that enters the bloodstream. Glucose is allowed into the cells via insulin so that the cells can use glucose as energy for body processes.

Insulin's role in metabolism is important. Insulin allows glucose to enter the muscle, fat, and liver cells, thus decreasing sugar in the blood. Insulin prompts the liver and muscle to store excess glucose as glycogen. Insulin can also regulate how much glucose the liver makes, thus shutting off production of glucose if needed. In the healthy person, all these hormone cascades should occur properly and in balance. It is when these functions teeter out of balance that problems arise.

Insulin resistance is potentially the most important item to be discussed when considering how to maintain improved blood sugar levels.

Insulin resistance occurs when the body makes insulin but is unable to utilize it effectively to maintain good blood sugar balance. When there is too much sugar in the blood over time, your insulin and pancreas become overworked compared to what the body was designed for. Because of this excess sugar, the body will often overproduce insulin at first. Then the body, noticing that there is excess insulin present, will increase its insulin receptors on the cells, allowing for more influx of sugar into the cells. This creates a problem. Now you have more sugar entering the cells than the body needs, thereby giving the cells an overload of sugar. Too much of a good thing is not always right. Functions of the cells are affected by this improper sugar and energy balance.

Over time, in someone who is insulin resistant, the sugars become harder to control and begin to creep up a bit higher than normal. Because of the regularly elevated blood sugars and consequently elevated insulin, the body gets used to this higher insulin level being needed to help control the blood sugar levels. The body literally cannot control its blood sugar without having higher amounts of insulin around, eventually causing islet-cell burnout in the pancreas. The insulin can no longer react the way it should, causing blood sugar levels to rise. After islet-cell burnout occurs, the body fails to produce the amount of insulin needed to control blood sugar levels. This is why it is so important to make sure that elevated blood glucose is treated as quickly as possible to prevent this serious complication. If untreated or unchanged, the inevitable end result of insulin resistance is type 2 diabetes mellitus. Insulin resistance is very difficult to treat once it sets in, and the longer someone has had insulin resistance, the longer it takes to reverse. Additionally, if the islet cells in the pancreas are burned out, it is difficult to rebuild or revitalize those cells to function well again.

Metabolic Syndrome

The term metabolic syndrome is often used synonymously with insulin resistance, but the two are a bit different. They occur so often together that they are often lumped into one. Not everyone with metabolic syndrome has insulin resistance, but many do. I think of metabolic syndrome as all the problems and symptoms that can come along with insulin resistance. For example, often metabolic syndrome is considered to be present when someone experiences three of the following:

- **elevated glucose levels**—fasting blood glucose level of 100 milligrams per deciliter (mg/dL) or above, or taking medication for elevated blood glucose
- **increased waist size**—waist measurement of 40 inches or more for men and 35 inches or more for women
- **elevated blood pressure (hypertension)**—blood pressure level of 130/85 or above, or taking medication for elevated blood pressure
- **elevated triglycerides in the blood**—triglyceride level of 150 mg/dL or above, or taking medication for elevated triglyceride level
- **poor lipid profiles in the blood such as high LDL with low HDL cholesterol**—HDL, the good cholesterol, level below 40 mg/dL for men and below 50 mg/dL for women, or taking medication for low HDL

The diagnosis of metabolic syndrome comes with a large set of increased morbidity risks. Metabolic syndrome is associated with increased risk for the following: obesity, cardiovascular disease, polycystic ovarian syndrome, chronic kidney disease, and nonalcoholic fatty liver disease.

Insulin resistance and type 2 diabetes both increase the function of an enzyme called aromatase, which converts testosterone to estradiol, a form of estrogen. Estrogen is a hormone that is seen in both male and female body chemistry and serves important functions.

This may not seem like a large deal, but it can explain some of the hormone imbalances that we see associated with insulin resistance or metabolic syndrome. Under the condition of higher estrogen, we see symptoms of estrogen dominance, including but not limited to increased risk for breast cancer. Interestingly, studies have shown that low testosterone increases the risk of developing type 2 diabetes and metabolic syndrome.

Sugar and cellular energy are also balanced by the amount of exercise you do. Energy ingested in the form of foods should equal the amount of energy used by the body for exercise plus the amount of energy needed for cellular processes. This is why exercise is so important. If you take away part of that equation, then you have a lot of energy going in in the form of food and then too much energy in the body that is essentially unusable. When the body has excess energy, it has to put it somewhere. Can you guess where that is? Yes, you guessed it, fat storage. If sugar metabolism is out of balance, then you will store a lot of your excess sugar as fat via conversion of your sugars into glycogen storage. This wasn't a problem in hunter-and-gathererer times because we didn't always have consistent meals, so when we did have a bigger meal, our bodies were meant to store it to get through times of eating lighter.

The current diet and lifestyle in most industrialized countries have taken away the need of the body to store energy, but, unfortunately, the body has not caught on and continues to store. This is why we see such a large epidemic of weight gain and obesity throughout our populations. It is my feeling that obesity is not by itself increasing people's risk for illnesses. I feel the sugar balance and insulin balance is off even before the weight gain begins. Obviously, insulin and sugar are not the only culprits as there are many other hormones that operate in balance together to create a healthy, vibrant organism.

The Freedom Diet is set up to be a 60-day program for jump-starting your road to recovery and better sugar balance and reduced mortality and morbidity risk. I will remind you, however, that changes made for health should be lifelong.

Glucose Problems in Nondiabetics

Prediabetes is a term used for people who have elevated blood sugar levels that are not high enough to qualify for diabetes. When someone has prediabetes, they are at extreme risk of developing diabetes and future cardiovascular complications such as stroke. This is the best time for someone to start making important changes in his or her life to reduce their risk of future diabetes and heart disease. Even before someone is diabetic, they should be working toward balanced health and blood sugar levels. Prediabetes just means that the person is going down the wrong path; if they don't change their habits, diabetes is nearly inevitable, because as we age, we have less homeostatic strength to keep hormones in optimal balance. Prolonged bad habits will always win against the aging body.

A hemoglobin A1c test is a good way to determine prediabetes. Hemoglobin is found in red blood cells, which carry oxygen throughout your body. When your blood sugar is not controlled (meaning that your blood sugar is too high), it builds up in your blood and combines with your hemoglobin, becoming "glycated." The HbA1c measures this glycated hemoglobin.

An HbA1c of 5.7 to 6.4 percent indicates prediabetes. People diagnosed with prediabetes may be retested in three months, six months, or one year. I retest people in three months so that we can better understand if our treatments and lifestyle changes are aggressive enough to reverse the disease process. People with an A1c below 5.7 percent may still be at risk for diabetes, depending on the presence of other characteristics that put them at risk, also known as risk factors. Risk factors include family history, sedentary lifestyle, high sugar consumption, and high fasting insulin. People with an A1c above 6.0 percent should be considered at very high risk of developing diabetes.

Fasting glucose can be another test used for diagnosing prediabetes. People with a fasting glucose level of 100 to 125 mg/dL have impaired fasting glucose or prediabetes. An oral glucose tolerance test (OGTT) can also be used to determine prediabetes, which involves drinking a sugary drink (containing 75 grams of glucose) after having fasted for at least eight hours and then testing the glucose two hours later. The OGTT can be used to diagnose diabetes, prediabetes, and gestational diabetes. If the two-hour blood glucose level from an OGTT is between 140 and 199 mg/dL, the person has a type of prediabetes called impaired glucose tolerance (IGT).

In short, nondiabetic individuals who cannot regulate their blood sugar levels are at an increased risk for developing diabetes. Most times medications are not recommended, as diet and exercise are the hallmark of how this stage should be treated. Without intervention a person is likely to develop diabetes within the next ten years. This can be an important stage at which to catch the problem. Since no medications are usually given at this time, it is important to start working really hard, because you certainly don't want to wait around for the diagnosis to catch up with you. Improving your insulin response will be really important, and one of the best ways to do that is to eliminate all sugars and most grains and lose weight. Exercise is also extremely effective at helping the body begin to regulate again. Some supplements can be very important as well.

How Do I Know If I Am Prediabetic?

There are certain signs that can tell you if you may have the chance of developing diabetes. One possible sign that you may be at risk of type 2 diabetes is darkened skin on certain parts of the body, a condition called acanthosis nigricans. Acanthosis nigricans can be a cutaneous sign of an underlying condition or disease. Acanthosis nigricans can commonly be seen on the neck, armpits, elbows, knees, and knuckles. It can be broken down into two forms, benign or malignant. It is rare that acanthosis is malignant. Benign types, sometimes described as "pseudoacanthosis nigricans," are much more common. The most common causes of acanthosis are obesity and insulin resistance. Another sign that you may acquire type 2 diabetes is developing a lot of skin tags. Look for these on the neck and around areas of your skin that rub against your clothing, such as bra or pant lines. And don't forget about the aforementioned blood sugar testing. A glucose tolerance test can be a great test to do before and after a strict diet and exercise regimen to understand how much progress you are making.

Diabetes

Diabetes is a disorder of metabolism in which your body simply cannot control the level of sugar that is in your blood. Diabetes affects many people in the United States each year and is listed as the seventh leading cause of death. The US Centers for Disease Control and Prevention (CDC) has predicted that 40 percent of Americans will develop diabetes in their lifetime. That is a significant number of the population and it absolutely can be prevented. In the United States, a new case of diabetes is diagnosed every 30 seconds; more than 1.9 million people are diagnosed each year.[37] Diabetes is also one of the most costly chronic illnesses. For example, Americans with diabetes incur medical expenses that are approximately 2.3 times higher than those incurred by Americans without diabetes.[38] The cost of caring for a diabetic child is significantly more than caring for a child without diabetes. Type 2 diabetes is a disease of improper diet and lifestyle. We are consuming too many items that have sugar in them for too many years. Our bodies were not designed to metabolize the amount of sugar we are consuming daily.

Diabetes complications include but are not limited to skin issues, eye complications such as glaucoma and cataracts, kidney disease, and neuropathy such as nerve damage to the lower extremities. Prolonged high blood glucose causes chemical changes in the nerves and causes damage to the blood vessels that bring important oxygen and nutrients to the nerves. In severe cases, neuropathy and circulation issues in the lower extremities can lead to amputation. Because diabetes affects the nerves, it is connected to an increased risk for many other conditions, such as stroke, high blood pressure, and gastroparesis, a condition in which your stomach takes too long to empty because it doesn't get the proper nerve stimulation it needs to function and digest properly. There are three main forms of diabetes. Diabetes insipidus is the least common form of diabetes and mainly involes the fluid balance in the body. Diabetes mellitus type 1 and type 2 are from an insulin deficiency and are much more common. A discussion of types 1 and 2 are below.

Diabetes Mellitus Type 1

Diabetes mellitus type 1 occurs when the body does not produce enough insulin. Remember that insulin is needed to remove glucose from the bloodstream and allow it back into the cell to give the cell energy. Research suggests that the cause behind the low insulin production in DM type 1 is lack of islet cell function or destruction of islet cells. Islet cells in the pancreas release insulin into circulation in the presence of elevated blood sugar. DM type 1 is an autoimmune disease. This means the destruction of the islet cells is occurring because the immune system is attacking the cells. This form of diabetes is treated with insulin due to the fact that the body simply cannot produce enough insulin to control the blood sugar levels. Improving the diet for a type 1 diabetic is still important and still therapeutic and should be done under the supervision of a primary care physician or endocrinologist.

Remember that all type 1 diabetics can live long, healthy, normal lives as long as they pay attention to their blood sugar levels and manage their insulin dosages appropriately. There is no reason that this cannot be tackled, and insulin doses kept at manageable levels by maintaining a healthy diet and lifestyle. Improving the diet by eliminating sugar and carbohydrate foods can improve DM type 1 significantly.

Diabetes Mellitus Type 2

Diabetes mellitus type 2 is the most common cause of diabetes. DM type 2 occurs when the body has prolonged elevated blood sugars, which puts the body into overdrive, causing it to produce more insulin on a regular basis in order to get all the sugar into the cells and out of the bloodstream. Eventually, all this up-regulation meets an end, and the pancreas can no longer keep up with the elevated blood sugar. DM type 2 is diagnosed by chronic elevated blood sugar levels. The same tests used to determine prediabetes are, not surprisingly, also used to test for DM type 2. These are: fasting blood sugar level, random blood sugar level, and a glycated hemoglobin, or HbA1c. If any one random blood sugar test is at or over 200 mg/dL, it is very suggestive of a diabetes diagnosis. Two separate fasting glucose readings at or over 126 mg/dL indicate a diabetes diagnosis. HbA1c over 6.5 percent at two different readings is also indicative of diabetes. Note that each of the test results indicating DM type 2 begins right at the top of the prediabetes threshold, making it obvious that prediabetes leads nowhere except to diabetes. An oral glucose tolerance (OGTT) test may also be performed. This can give us a good idea of how someone is adapting to their blood sugar levels and how well their insulin is working. If confirmed by a second test, a two-hour glucose level of 200 mg/dL or above means a person has diabetes. In some cases, to help determine insulin efficiency, insulin as well as glucose can be checked periodically two hours postprandial (after the patient has ingested the sugar solution).

We do understand that diabetes has a strong genetic family history. Although we haven't pinpointed specific genes to explain how this disease is inherited, I suppose we can theorize that epigenetics has a large amount to do with it.

Epigenetics

Epigenetics is complicated, but I will give some basics here. There are many diseases that are inheritable, but not necessarily based on a particular DNA sequence. We understand that the environment in which the DNA exists and thrives has significant impact on how the genes are expressed. For example, there have been studies involving genetic identical twins who were raised in different environments and then grow to express different disease risks. We know they have the exact same DNA sequences, but somehow some genes were turned off and some were turned on. This also is shown with the developing fetus. We understand that when the developing fetus is exposed to various stressors, such as environmental stressors, hormonal imbalances, nutritional deficiencies, and drug exposures, it has a direct effect on how the genetics of that baby will be expressed. We understand that drug- and alcohol-affected children may likely have more issues than babies born to a "clean" mom.

How epigenetics may come into play with diabetes is that when parents with diabetes have children and grandchildren, sometimes the stage has been set for the expression of certain genes. If those children are fed a high-sugar diet, they are almost destined to turn out like their parents and develop diabetes. Sometimes, though, even after putting a child into a healthy environment, if there have been generations of genetic expression, it can be hard to shut those genes off or prevent them from triggering the diabetic insulin/sugar issue.

MTHFR Defect

Speaking of genetics, there are many genetic defects that can affect our health. How the body stimulates its enzymes to function can be affected by various genetic mutations that affect methylation.

DNA methylation is a biochemical process whereby a methyl group is added to the cytosine or adenine DNA nucleotides. Methylation of DNA is balanced with acetylation, and this causes important genes to be highlighted or silenced. This balance is critical. MTHFR mutations are well-researched genetic defects that may play an important role in diabetes and the evaluation of many chronic health issues. MTHFR is a gene that codes for methylenetetrahydrofolate reductase, an enzyme that plays an important role in folate metabolism. Folate, or folic acid, in turn plays a vital role in DNA synthesis.

Genetic abnormalities occur when a base of the DNA is switched with a different base. Base compounds are found in pairs because two strands of DNA wind together via weak chemical bonds to form a double helix. A base pair is two chemical bases bonded to one another, forming a rung of the DNA ladder. The DNA molecule consists of two strands that wind around each other like a twisted ladder. Each strand has a backbone made of alternating sugar (deoxyribose) and phosphate groups. Attached to each sugar is one of four bases—adenine (A), cytosine (C), guanine (G), or thymine (T). The two strands are held together by hydrogen bonds between the bases, with adenine forming a base pair with thymine, and cytosine forming a base pair with guanine.[39]

As with any genetic inheritance, you will get one copy of a gene from your mom and one copy of the same gene from your dad. Therefore someone can get a normal copy from one parent and an abnormal copy from the opposite parent, which we call a *heterozygous state*. A more significant abnormality occurs when a "bad" copy is inherited from both mom and dad. When this occurs, we consider this state to be homozygous. *Homozygous* would also refer to someone who inherited normal copies from both mom and dad. Because the MTHFR defect can negatively affect folate synthesis, this can affect methylation reactions such as the conversion from homocysteine to methionine. Medical literature has connected elevated homocysteine to increased risk for cardiovascular disease, which is the leading cause of death in people with diabetes and also the leading cause of death among Americans. Elevated homocysteine has been shown to be associated with cardiovascular disease, atherosclerosis, stroke, and deep vein thrombosis or clotting. This clotting can also affect pregnancies and can be associated with miscarriages due to the clotting in the arteries that lead to the placenta, causing decreased blood flow to the fetus.

The MTHFR enzyme is important in many other reactions in the body, especially those that balance neurotransmitter activity in the nervous system. It plays a role in the balance of serotonin, dopamine, and norepinephrine. We also find MTHFR function related to histamine balance, SAMe (an important methyl donor within the body), and glutathione, referred to as GSH. GSH is a very important antioxidant in the body. In fact, it is one of the main antioxidant drivers in the body, conducting the complex process of helping the body reduce oxidative stress reactions and improve detoxification.

Although we understand quite a few genetic defects that occur within the human genome, genetic abnormalities are largely uncommon compared with the significant number of genes that are put together correctly in the body. When a gene is large, it has a larger potential for defects to occur. The MTHFR gene is a rather large genetic sequence. There are many variations that have been noted in the MTHFR gene, but we are only beginning to understand some of the main variations. The MTHFR genes that have been studied the most are referred to as the C677T MTHFR gene mutation and the A1298C MTHFR gene mutation. The numbers relate to where in the gene the genetic alteration, or abnormality, occurs, and the letters are the bases involved.

The C677T MTHFR defect has been studied extensively, and both homozygous and heterozygous abnormalities can have significant implications on methylation. How I describe methylation to my patients is the ability to balance the methylation of DNA with acetylation. DNA needs to be methylated and acetylated to stay in balance. An excess of one or the other results in either overmethylation or undermethylation. The C677T MTHFR defect can result in up to 70 percent improper MTHFR enzyme function, potentially affecting many body processes, like those listed above.

The A1298C MTHFR defect has been shown to have an effect on the MTHFR enzyme, but hasn't been found to be as significantly associated with decreased enzyme function unless the abnormality is found to be homozygous. Because of its more mild effect, a heterozygous abnormality in this gene hasn't been found to be as significant as defects in the 677 area of the MTHFR gene.

MTHFR Testing

MTHFR testing has become increasingly common. It is a simple blood test that can be ordered from most laboratories. The two main MTHFR defects that are tested are the C677T and the A1298C. Test results will look like one of the following below. Having normal genetic sequences for both will result in normal function of the MTHFR enzyme. Consequently, on the other end of the spectrum, having homozygous abnormalities of both will result in significant decreases of the MTHFR enzyme function with resulting heightened methylation issues.

677 C/C: homozygous normal copies
677 C/T: heterozygous abnormality
677 T/T: homozygous abnormality
1298 A/A: homozygous normal copies
1298 A/C: heterozygous abnormality
1298 C/C: homozygous abnormality

MTHFR and Diabetes

While MTHFR gene mutations do not directly cause diabetes, undermethylation and elevated homocysteine (which can be caused by MTHFR) are serious risk factors in the development of type 2 diabetes. In a recent study, the MTHFR 677 TT genotype was associated with DM type 2 susceptibility and complications such as diabetic retinopathy, diabetic polyneuropathy, and ischemic heart disease. The MTHFR 1298 CC and AC genotypes were associated with diabetic retinopathy and diabetic polyneuropathy. Additionally, long-term exposure to homocysteine causes issues with insulin secretions, cell death, and beta cell metabolism, which can lead to insulin resistance, underproduction of insulin, and elevated glucose.

Diabetic patients often suffer from low glutathione, GSH. This can be a result of prolonged hyperglycemia or an MTHFR defect. Uncontrolled diabetes can reduce the availability of GSH precursors, therefore offering less substrate on which to make GSH. GSH is a very important antioxidant and is important in diminishing free-radical damage in the body. Diabetes type 2 is increasingly being connected with low-level inflammation within the body and immune system imbalance. For example, we understand that people with diabetes are more susceptible to some infections. Low GSH will only compound this risk, not offering the antioxidant protection the body needs during antigen exposure.

As we already understand, diabetic peripheral neuropathy can be an unpleasant complication of diabetes and can result in discomfort, extremity lesions, pain and paresthesias, and even amputation of limbs. Another study published by the National Institutes of Health confirms a strong relationship between diabetic peripheral neuropathy and defects in the 677 position of the MTHFR gene.[41]

Can You Change MTHFR?

Unfortunately, the MTHFR defect will not change, as you inherit it when you are conceived. Unlike blood pressure and blood sugar, the MTHFR status of a person will not change with treatment. But understanding your methylation status and speaking to your doctor about it can help you formulate a treatment plan that you can use lifelong to combat the methylation issues you may have.

Diabetes Type 3 Is Really Alzheimer's?

You may or may not have heard of anyone discussing diabetes type 3. I wanted to bring this to your awareness in case you hear it in the future. Essentially, diabetes type 3 is Alzheimer's disease. We understand now that Alzheimer's can be related to the MTHFR gene. Even as early as 2008, describing Alzheimer's as a diabetes-related disease was confirmed in the *Journal of Diabetes Science and Technology*. The report concluded that the term "type 3 diabetes" accurately represents Alzheimer's disease, and further concluded that Alzheimer's disease is a form of diabetes that affects the brain, mimicking the molecular and biochemical processes seen in both type 1 and type 2 diabetes.[42]

Alzheimer's was first described in 1905 by a German psychiatrist who performed an autopsy on a woman who had early cognitive decline. He was the first person to describe what we understand now as the hallmark of Alzheimer's, amyloid plaques. Amyloid plaques are protein buildups of tangled cell fragments. Amyloid plaques are still being used to diagnose Alzheimer's disease. Up to one-third of adults experience some form of dementia or Alzheimer's by the time they reach the age of 85.[43]

It has been over a hundred years since we have discovered this disease, and there hasn't been significant success in reducing Alzheimer's or formulating a treatment to ward off or treat its effects. Alzheimer's is still very poorly understood. There are many theories about why Alzheimer's disease has developed, including theories of high inflammatory states, oxidative stressors, metal metabolism problems, deficient enzymes, and blood sugar levels and diabetes, as well as others. It is most likely to be a combination of many of these issues.

Diabetic Medications
Insulin

As mentioned, insulin is a hormone that the body produces to help manage blood sugar levels. It allows the entrance of sugar into cells and out of the bloodstream. Sometimes, individuals are dependent upon an outside source of insulin. Insulin is available in various forms and most involve the patient making small injections with a short needle into their subcutaneous tissue, underneath the skin. Insulin can be given by a syringe, injection pen, or an insulin pump. An insulin pump is a little different in that the person doesn't have to actually inject the insulin because it stays fixed to the skin and allows a continuous flow of insulin to be delivered to the body. All type 1 diabetics will have to use insulin for the rest of their lives because their pancreas is no longer doing a good job of producing the amount of insulin their body needs. Depending on their health and diligence, the insulin doses for type 1 diabetics range drastically. Again, I repeat that healthy diet and lifestyle choices can help even type 1 diabetics lose weight, feel better, and reduce their insulin doses. All type 1 diabetics undergoing a major diet change should visit with their physician to discuss the diet as well as future insulin monitoring.

Some type 2 diabetics also become dependent on insulin for various reasons. One reason this occurs is because they have tried medications and other means to control the blood sugar, but it remains high. Often, if they continue to eat sugary foods, consume alcohol, and live in excess stress with poor exercise habits, their blood sugar continues to spiral out of control until they need insulin to help keep it regulated.

The article "What Is Insulin?" notes that various types of insulin are used to treat diabetes. They include:

- Rapid-acting insulin: It starts working approximately 15 minutes after injection and peaks at approximately one hour but continues to work for two to four hours. This is usually taken before a meal and in addition to a long-acting insulin.
- Short-acting insulin: It starts working approximately 30 minutes after injection and peaks at approximately two to three hours but will continue to work for three to six hours. It is usually given before a meal and in addition to a long-acting insulin.
- Intermediate-acting insulin: It starts working approximately two to four hours after injection and peaks approximately four to twelve hours later and continues to work for 12–18 hours. It is usually taken twice a day and in addition to a rapid- or short-acting insulin.
- Long-acting insulin: It starts working several hours after injection and works for approximately twenty-four hours. If necessary, it is used in combination with rapid- or short-acting insulin.[44]

Metformin

Metformin, also referred to as Glucophage, is a very commonly prescribed medication for type 2 diabetes. Metformin is used to treat elevated blood sugar levels that are not controlled by the body. It can be used alone or in combination with other blood-sugar-lowing medications or insulin. For metformin to do its job properly, the amount you take must be balanced against the amount and type of food you eat and the amount of exercise you do. Metformin works by decreasing the amount of glucose released from the liver. This is extremely important because if we can reduce the glucose that comes from the liver, then the body will only have the burden of controlling the blood sugar rise from eating. Therefore, dietary changes while on metformin can be extremely effective and can help someone get off metformin in the future.

When you start this diet and exercise plan, if you are on metformin, you will initially want to test your blood sugar often to find out if it is too low. You may want to consult your physician about medication changes if you are regularly experiencing low blood sugar. It is best to have your doctor help reduce your dose rather than relying on consuming more sugar to bring your blood sugar back up to normal.

Metformin's list of potential drug interactions is significant, as is the list of potential side effects. Side effects may include bloating, gas, diarrhea, upset stomach, and loss of appetite. It should be taken with food to minimize symptoms. In rare cases, lactic acidosis may occur in people with abnormal kidney or liver function. It is not often that metformin causes low blood sugar. Interestingly, I have had a handful of patients who were having a hard time controlling their blood sugar on metformin and decided to stop taking it. Miraculously, their blood sugars stabilized better on our treatment plan after they stopped taking it compared to when they were taking it. I can't explain why this has happened, but I have noted it more than once.

Because type 2 diabetes can often be controlled through diet and lifestyle changes, if you have not started this medication yet, please follow the Freedom Diet and lifestyle changes first, because most likely you will not need the metformin after that. It is always important to improve health through diet and lifestyle when you can, number one, to reduce the amount of pharmaceutical medications you are on, and number two, because when you work on improving a particular health concern by changing your diet and lifestyle, then so many other things get better as well. For example, taking up exercise and improving your diet to improve your blood pressure also improves your energy, sleep, cardiovascular risk, and so on.

Metformin is also used in insulin resistance and polycystic

ovarian syndrome. Although it is not FDA-approved for the latter, many physicians prescribe it to help women improve their insulin response. Again, I point out that changing the insulin response takes time, but can be managed without the use of pharmaceutical medications.

Additionally, drugs like metformin may increase homocysteine levels in people with MTHFR C677T mutations. So it is especially important that people with diabetes test and treat their MTHFR enzyme function.

Farxiga

We can't assume that all pharmaceuticals are safe and effective just because a physician is prescribing them. For example, a newer drug approved by the FDA in December of 2013, Farxiga, has been documented to have many adverse side effects. Farxiga is not recommended for patients with type 1 diabetes or patients with increased ketones in their urine or blood. It is contraindicated in patients who have moderate or severe kidney impairment, end-stage renal disease, or who are on dialysis. In fact, in 2012, the FDA didn't want to approve the drug originally because they didn't feel there was enough information about its benefits and risks. The most common side effects from this drug are genital fungal infections such as yeast infection and urinary tract infections. There were enough documented cases of bladder cancer for the FDA to be concerned. Trials revealed that patients taking the drug were five times more likely to develop bladder cancer and twice as likely to get breast cancer. Diana Zuckerman, president of the National Research Center for Women & Families, had serious concerns about the safety of this medication. She wrote in February of 2014, "The agency just approved a new diabetes medication that doesn't noticeably improve health but may in fact cause cancer."[45] Who knows what changed the regulators' minds between 2012 and 2013, but I am sure that some of you can guess. They say now that they approved it but are making sure that trials and tests continue through its use. Hopefully we don't find out that it may be too late for some people for whom the risks clearly outweighed the benefits.

The Diet and Lifestyle Prescription

There are many glucose-control medications on the market other than insulin and metformin. Some medications may be beneficial at reducing blood sugar levels, but all come with the potential for adverse side effects. Positive diet and lifestyle changes don't come with negative side effects. Actually, the only side effect of this diet and lifestyle intervention method is freedom—the freedom to do some of the things you have not been able to do in a long time.

My theory on medication is that when you try to just take a medication to cure an ailment, the philosophy behind the prescription is all wrong. Just taking cholesterol medication for high cholesterol while not changing your diet and lifestyle doesn't decrease your mortality risk from having a heart attack. The same can be said about taking a diabetic medication without changing your diet. If you are not reducing sugar in your diet or incorporating better lifestyle changes and are instead simply depending on a pharmaceutical medication to do the work, eventually either the medication will fail, you will develop side effects, or other parts of your body will start to develop problems. The "diet and lifestyle prescription" in this book should be viewed as an orange bottle with a white lid. It is something that is being prescribed for your ailment and it should be adhered to daily, just like you would take a medication daily.

I am not saying that you should quit all your current medications, but I am saying that the medications you take are going to be more effective or eventually not needed if you change your habits now. Medications can be used as a bridge from your old life to your new one. Maybe they make you and your doctor feel more comfortable as you transition into a better lifestyle and diet. As mentioned previously, when you change your diet and lifestyle to affect one health issue, many health issues are addressed. For example, I have many patients who come to see me for asthma, elevated cholesterol, elevated blood pressure, elevated sugar, and various other issues. When we incorporate diet and lifestyle changes along with supplements for these patients, many of their other complaints resolve also. We have had many patients who come in for help with weight or blood sugar issues, we put them on a program, and when they return, they are also sleeping better, they have better energy, and their back pain has improved. Sometimes these are things they hadn't even mentioned in their initial visit.

What we need to remember is that the body always works as a whole, and it should always be approached that way. When we see patients, instead of addressing their complaints one by one, we should step across the street and look at them with a different perspective. I want to get a better view of what is happening to them on the inside and how their body works, how it processes toxicity, and how it will adapt to a diet and lifestyle change. When the body is approached as a whole, incredible life-changing things happen quickly. We have had numerous patients on metformin or another blood-sugar-regulating medication who adopted a healthier diet and were still struggling with the control of their blood sugar. We have had to brainstorm why this is. Why would the blood sugar control get worse in some patients on medications when they adopted a healthier diet? My assumption is that as we begin to control the diet, the actual control of sugar balance and insulin is clouded by the pharmaceutical medication. It doesn't allow the body to begin balancing the sugar on its own. If we can determine that patients are following our diet strictly, then often taking that patient off of their blood-sugar-controlling medication actually normalizes their blood sugars.

I am bringing this point up now so that if you start this program and have difficulty balancing your blood sugars, you will know that you need to return to your physician to have a conversation about your medication. Most people show improvements in regulation and lowering of their resting glucose levels as they start this diet, but there are some who will have numbers that fluctuate more. If you are one of the people who are fluctuating too much, meet with your doctor to discuss your next steps.

List of Diabetic Medications by Purpose

Different medications serve different purposes. This is why many individuals will be on several medications for the same illness. This is true of diabetes medications. Below is a list of diabetic medications and the purpose they are supposed to serve. The generic name is listed first, followed by common brand names in parenthesis:

- **Decreases the amount of glucose released by the liver**
  - » Metformin (Glucophage)
- **Stimulates the pancreas to release more insulin, both right after a meal and then over several hours**
  - » Glyburide (Diabeta, Micronase)
  - » Glipizide (Glucotrol, Glucotrol XL)
  - » Glimepiride (Amaryl)
- **Stimulates the pancreas to release more insulin right after a meal**
  - » Repaglinide (Prandin)
  - » Nateglinide (Starlix)
- **Makes the body more sensitive to the effects of insulin**
  - » Rosaglitazine (Avandia) a thiazolidinedione
  - » Pioglitazone (Actos)
- **Improves insulin level after a meal and lowers the amount of glucose made by the body**
  - » Sitagliptin (Januvia)
  - » Saxagliptin (Onglyza)
  - » Linagliptin (Tradjenta)
- **Slows the absorption of carbohydrates into the bloodstream after eating**
  - » Acarbose (Precose)
  - » Miglitol (Glyset)
- **Works with other diabetes medications to lower blood glucose**
  - » Colesevelam (Welchol)

Side Effects

Here are just some of the side effects one might expect if they took one or more of the medications listed above: gas, diarrhea, stomach discomfort, sore throat, stuffy nose, upper respiratory infection, interference with levothyroxine (a very common thyroid medication), edema (fluid retention), occasional skin rash, irritability. We are continuing to prescribe these medications by the boatload to Americans who are overweight and diabetic. Why not just talk to these people about diet and lifestyle changes? Why do we continue to be owned by pharmaceutical companies?

CHAPTER 5

Blood Sugar and Its Relation to Inflammation

Current Diet Leads to Elevated Blood Sugar and Health Issues

As discussed in depth earlier, the way we are eating has detrimental effects on our health, including our balance of blood sugar, or blood glucose. Even if we are able to keep our blood glucose levels balanced while consuming large amounts of sugar, we are burning out our resources much too quickly to continue living healthily for a long period of time. Oftentimes, even if someone is not eating the obvious sugar sources such as sweetened drinks, pastries, cookies, cakes, and candy, other quick sources of sugar can eventually cause detriment to the important homeostatic mechanisms in the body. For example, consuming a lot of white rice, pasta, bread, alcohol, and potatoes can have a huge impact on blood sugar balance and the ability to maintain stable levels of blood glucose and insulin long-term. Additionally, drinking juice daily while not consuming enough fiber can have an impact on long-term blood glucose balance. These food items turn into instant sugar when consumed and present a larger glycemic insult to the system, requiring a more robust insulin response to regulate blood glucose. Eating these sugary and starchy items regularly will eventually strain the system enough to cause a prediabetic or diabetic situation. This is why so many people are diagnosed with diabetes and why the diabetes epidemic continues to increase. Diabetes currently affects more than 387 million people worldwide and is expected to affect 592 million by 2035.[46] We are not doing enough to reverse this disease manifestation in our population, and marketers who are putting sugary food items on the shelves in grocery stores are not helping. They are only concerned about their bottom line—not the consumer's health.

Consuming foods that trigger inflammation will continue to promote ill health. Inflammatory triggers in the gastrointestinal tract will cause significant imbalances in the way the immune system functions and can trigger a body-wide inflammatory attack. Elevated inflammation levels are connected to most chronic illnesses worldwide. We understand inflammation and its health implications much better than we did 10 to 20 years ago, but are we taking great strides to change what is on the supermarket shelves? Are we paying attention to inflammatory food triggers to ensure we bring in adequate nutrients and avoid foods that can confuse the gastrointestinal tract lining? As mentioned earlier, the homeostasis of the immune system is based on the health of the gut lining, which depends on many attributes for its proper function. For example, consuming appropriate amounts of fiber, obtaining nutrients in the form of vegetables, and avoiding artificially flavored or sweetened food will all promote a better gastrointestinal tract lining and thereby promote better nutrient absorption and decreased inflammation potential. Additionally, maintaining proper probiotic balance will help to promote better digestion and absorption of nutrients and will help to preserve the immune presence at the GI border, which is important in balancing the inflammation cascade.

Elevated Sugar Is Connected to Diabetes and Kidney Disease

Any long-term elevation of blood glucose leads to diabetes. Don't fool yourself by thinking that upward-creeping blood sugar won't ever develop into diabetes. I have some patients who have a blood sugar of 115 or 120, and because it doesn't fit the diabetes diagnosis, I can't motivate them to cut out the sugar. I can't get them to understand the implications of having a blood sugar level that high. As much as I try to stress prevention, some people don't get it. I am here to inspire you to get it. Understand that elevated blood glucose is not getting you anywhere positive. You are going down the wrong road if you allow blood sugar levels to continue rising, inching you toward a diabetes diagnosis. In 2011, diabetes was the leading cause of kidney failure, nontraumatic lower-limb amputations, and new cases of blindness among adults in the United States.[47]

Elevated Sugar Is Connected to Cardiovascular Complications

Heart disease is the number-one killer of both men and women in the world. Many health complications precede cardiovascular disease, and blood sugar is definitely one of them. Inflammation is stimulated by various health problems, as discussed earlier. Elevated blood sugar has a direct connection to oxidative stress and inflammation. Oxidative stress and inflammation are the backbone of heart disease and its complications. Diabetes is a major cause of heart disease and stroke.[48]

Cooking Foods All Wrong

Diabetes has become a worldwide epidemic. With diabetes-related morbidity and mortality increasing each year, the disease is causing a significant impact on our health care system. Of special note is advanced research on the way we cook foods and its connection to inflammation and oxidative stress.

AGEs

AGEs, advanced glycation end products, or glycotoxins, lead to advanced or accelerated aging. You can think about glycotoxins as compounds in your body that have too much sugar stuck to them, rendering them more harmful than helpful. AGEs present a "cute" acronym because of how intimately connected to AGING they are. Simply put, AGEs accelerate aging via inflammation, oxidative damage, and the "sugarization" of important molecules in the body. The more AGEs you accumulate, the faster you will age. AGEs are made endogenously (within the body) and are also accumulated exogenously (through diet). We have control over both endogenous and exogenous AGEs.

AGEs are formed when glucose binds to amino acids and lipids in the body. Endogenous AGEs form in the presence of prolonged elevated blood sugar. Exogenous AGEs, found in many animal products that are high in protein and fat, can be increased through various cooking methods. Dry cooking methods such as grilling, toasting, broiling, roasting, and browning of animal products are directly related to higher dietary AGEs. Heating animal products in this manner increases AGEs significantly, often by tenfold compared to the heating of fruits and vegetables! This browning reaction, called the Maillard reaction, results in AGE production. Even that pretty brown piece of toast you just made has increased its AGE content. The more cooked the item of food you eat, the more AGEs you are consuming.

AGEs are very damaging chemicals. AGEs cause oxidative damage, and in turn oxidative damage increases formation of more AGEs, presenting your body with another vicious cycle that is difficult to beat. Some AGE formation is reversible, but the longer an AGE exists in the body, the more potential it has to form an irreversible compound. When AGEs are elevated to an irreversible point, they linger in our blood for a long time and begin to cause damage. Many times this damage occurs to blood vessels, causing stiffening and deterioration which eventually leads to cardiovascular disease, our nation's number-one fatal illness. An overabundance of AGEs also leads to increased inflammation, kidney damage, Alzheimer's disease, diabetes, and many other chronic illnesses. A good way to think about AGEs is as proteins that are "sugarized" within the body. Remember the hemoglobin A1c we discussed, which is checked to diagnose and monitor diabetes. A glycated hemoglobin is one example of an AGE in the body. It is hemoglobin, a protein, being sugarized (because there is excess sugar in the bloodstream), and that is why we are able to use it to monitor diabetes. You can monitor how much AGE you are producing or consuming by monitoring your HbA1c levels. Consider that if your hemoglobin is glycated then many of your other proteins are glycated as well. Dietary causes of diabetes such as exogenous AGEs have been overlooked in the treatment of diabetic individuals. Avoiding sugary foods is only one dietary suggestion. Other dietary suggestions should be included during the doctor–patient visit, including avoiding the Maillard reaction when cooking animal products, and increasing vegetables and fruits while decreasing overall consumption of animal products.

CHAPTER 6

Obesity

The Causes of Obesity

Obesity is not just a problem of eating too much and not exercising enough. Medical researchers simply don't know enough about the complexity of obesity. We understand on a large scale obesity's health implications. We understand that obesity is directly linked to inflammation, heart disease, increased cancer risk, and increased all-cause mortality. This means that obese patients will have a greater risk of dying than their thinner comrades. Obesity is a worldwide epidemic. A 2013 analysis of the Global Burden of Disease reported in the *Lancet* that between 1980 and 2013, the combined prevalence of overweight and obesity worldwide rose by 27.5 percent in adults and 47.1 percent in children.[49]

Obesity is triggered and controlled by more than increased calories and not enough exercise. Obesity also has a genetic component, in addition to insulin resistance problems, hormone balance and regulation problems, mental–emotional triggers, and so much more.

Obesity is a part of the metabolic syndrome, which was discussed in chapter 4. Metabolic syndrome is diagnosed by a set of criteria that include abdominal obesity or abnormal weight, insulin resistance, dyslipidemia, and hypertension. Individuals with metabolic syndrome face increased risk for type 2 diabetes and cardiovascular diseases.

Obesity is very multifaceted, and at the root of the problem lies the overall hormone balance within the body, one of the most important factors in the progression of obesity. When I say hormones, I know that you will think about the sex hormones like estrogen, progesterone, and testosterone, but don't forget that insulin is a hormone and therefore very important in the development of obesity. To better understand obesity from a hormone perspective, imagine that you have a complex interplay of hormones working to either store fat or bring it out of circulation while also trying to deal with the type and amount of calories you are eating and how much you are burning while working out. The hormones are in a constant flux, responding appropriately or inappropriately to all situations, including mental and emotional stress, physical stress, environmental stressors, improper dieting strategies, and so on.

In addition, hormone balance is the most important factor in how an obese body will respond to treatment. If we can optimize the hormone balance of an individual, then the treatments we suggest will work better quicker. I say quicker, but I want to clarify that treatment of an obese person is lifelong and can be a slow endeavor. A lot of learned behaviors can be present in someone with health problems, including someone with obesity. Additionally, when the body is used to functioning a certain way for a long period of time, it becomes its homeostasis, and even though we think it is out of balance, the body does not because that particular way of doing things has become the status quo. Sometimes it is a long process of "retraining" the body to think differently, "retraining" the hormones to act a little differently, and trying our best to improve receptor-site response by decreasing oxidative stress and inflammation.

Actually, the treatment of anything should be lifelong. As soon as we stop weeding our garden, it begins to grow the wrong plants—weeds—displacing the plants we want. The same is true with the body. We must continue to weed and water our garden always. Another analogy I use to describe this to my new patients is that we are starting by turning the boat around. It has been drifting downstream, and now we want to start going back upstream. This process is often difficult. It is hard to turn the boat around initially, especially if it is a very large boat. The larger the boat, or body, the more effort we have to put into it to turn things around. But once we get going, it will be a bit easier, keeping in mind that once you are headed back upstream, you will always have to keep rowing. The minute you stop, you start letting the current take you back downstream again.

Working on your health is a permanent task.

Leptin Control

I want to mention some of the other important hormones involved in obesity. Obesity interventions should include more than just calorie restriction and exercise. The interventions that are going to work will involve lifestyle interventions and supplements that also affect the basic biochemistry of the patient. Making sure that insulin resistance is decreasing, making sure that hormones are functioning properly but are also being broken down properly, and ensuring a better-balanced symphony of hormone function is important.

Leptin is one of the best-known hormone markers for obesity, and we understand that it has effects on multiple organ systems. Nearly universally, leptin is low in obese individuals. Altered leptin signaling often occurs in obesity and can lead to an array of cardiovascular complications. One of the main jobs of leptin is to control the amount of calories consumed by a person. It tells the central nervous system (the brain and spinal cord) how much energy (calories) has been consumed. If someone has just consumed a meal, then leptin will communicate that it has an abundance of energy stores, thereby reducing appetite and restricting more food intake. Leptin will then initiate energy expenditure in the body. Absence of leptin will result in improper satiety and can lead to increased appetite and increased food consumption. This may result from the disruption of leptin communication and control in the hypothalamus. The hypothalamus plays a significant role in balancing many hormones in the body and creating the "set point" your body wants to maintain for weight.

The lack of leptin also has significant cardiovascular ramifications. It is connected to hypertension, congestive heart failure, atherosclerosis, depressed myocardial contractile function, fatty acid metabolism, and can be connected to ischemia problems like stroke or heart attack.[50]

Adiponectin

Adiponectin is a collagen-like plasma protein hormone. It is secreted by adipocytes (fat cells). Low levels of adiponectin are associated with insulin resistance, diabetes, atherosclerosis, and coronary artery disease.[51] Adiponectin helps someone maintain healthy weight by helping the body process glucose and balance the insulin response. There are natural ways to increase adiponectin levels, such as increasing the intake of monounsaturated fats and other healthy fats, like omega-3 fatty acids, and exercising. It is easy to check fasting adiponectin levels at your next blood draw. This could be a fun marker for you to check before and after this 60-day program.

CHAPTER 7

The Hormone Symphony

We've talked briefly about hormones and how they function in regard to diabetes, obesity, and other health factors, but what is important to know is that you have a whole symphony of hormones in various states of function. You have some hormones that are currently active and other hormones that have just finished their job and are being taken back out of circulation. You also have hormones in the start pen, patiently waiting to be stimulated for use.

There are a significant number of hormones in the body that turn processes on and off, open gates and channels within cell membranes for transport of molecules in and out, and perform various other complicated functions. Hormones control metabolism, immune response, blood sugar balance, blood pressure balance, mood, sleep, digestion, appetite, growth, feeling of connection with others, milk production during lactation, and so on. It is impossible in a short chapter to list all the bodily functions that are controlled by hormones. Optimizing hormone control, then, becomes extremely important in reducing chronic illness, improving blood sugar levels, controlling inflammation, reducing or slowing the aging process, improving blood chemistry and lipid levels, and preventing chronic illness.

Hormones are researched for their vast array of duties in relationship to many illnesses. There are various hormones that are studied more extensively in relationship to cardiovascular health. Remember, cardiovascular disease is almost a sure complication of diabetes, but also a very common complication in nondiabetics as well. We'll discuss some of these hormones below.

Hypothalamus, the Director

The hypothalamus works in unison with the pituitary and other glands to form the body's "set point" for weight. The longer you are at a particular weight, the more the body begins to adapt to that particular weight as its set point. This is an important concept to understand because many people are doing what I consider yo-yo dieting. Although I think some dieting is necessary in order for some people to lose weight, I feel that the maintenance program is more important than the weight-loss program itself. Therefore, I suggest that if you work really hard and lose 20 pounds, you take at least two to three months after the weight loss to continue working at keeping the 20 pounds off. If you can do this, you are more likely to stay at your new "set point" as long as you keep your habits healthy.

The hypothalamus is a gland in the brain that is involved in linking the pituitary to the endocrine system, thereby allowing communication between the nervous system and the endocrine system. The nervous system can be thought of as the brain, spinal cord, and all of the neurological processes that occur as part of nervous system homeostasis. The endocrine system is a complex system of glands that secrete various hormones into the blood to carry out biological processes within the body. These hormones are secreted by endocrine glands with the direct goal of reaching receptor sites at distant organs and carrying out a particular function. The pineal gland, pituitary gland, pancreas, ovaries, testes, thyroid gland, parathyroid gland, hypothalamus, gastrointestinal tract, and adrenal glands are the main endocrine organs.

As you can imagine, the endocrine system has a huge effect on how the body functions as a whole and what major diseases it may become susceptible to. Poor endocrine function, even at just one of those glands, will affect the other glands. Poor stimulation of the gland itself can cause a whole host of problems. Poor receptor-site function for particular hormones can also create trouble. A good example of this is insulin resistance, in which insulin receptors have become blunted in their response to insulin, thereby needing more insulin to do their job. The hypothalamus's job is complex. It makes and secretes many hormones that stimulate the many important endocrine glands. I consider it the director of the symphony, as it is integral to the functioning and balance of all the other hormones.

Pituitary, the Mother

The pituitary gland is about the size of a small pea and sits right in the center of the head, behind the bridge of the nose. It consists of two parts, the posterior pituitary and the anterior pituitary. The posterior pituitary has one main job, regulating the balance of fluid in the body by secreting a hormone called antidiuretic hormone.

The anterior pituitary is another director of sorts. It still takes a lot of its direction from the hypothalamus but plays an intimate role in controlling many of the glands important in the sex hormone cascade, thyroid balance, and adrenal gland function. Additionally, the anterior pituitary makes growth hormone, an important hormone associated with growth and sleep. It decreases significantly in the aging population. Growth hormone deficiency can easily be seen in the elderly, who begin to have what we consider jowls. Jowls are seen when the lower part of a person's cheeks begins to sag.

The anterior pituitary is the main secretor of stimulatory hormones that direct distant glands to function appropriately, managing the multitude of hormones working together to form an intricate network of signaling and feedback mechanisms. The pituitary is also very important in lactation and our feeling of connection with others through the secretion of a hormone called oxytocin. Oxytocin is important in our feeling of connectedness to our social circles, families, and those around us. Interestingly, having an emotional connection to a clan, group, or family is related to improved health. And lack of a significant other has been directly linked to increased risk for heart disease.

Thyroid, the Protector

Is your thyroid functioning optimally? Yes, it comes back normal on a blood test, but does that mean that the levels of your thyroid hormone are optimal and doing what they are supposed to be doing to trigger proper metabolism? I always speak about the thyroid being the battery of the body, but the most common complaint that I see in my office from every type of patient is fatigue. What is happening to our batteries?

Here are some thyroid-deficiency symptoms that can alert you to the fact that your thyroid may not be functioning optimally. These symptoms may suggest hypothyroidism, or underfunctioning of the thyroid:

- sensitive to cold
- cold hands and feet
- puffy eyes and/or puffy face in the morning
- difficulty getting out of bed in the morning
- feeling more tired when at rest rather than during activity
- dry skin and hair
- hair loss
- constipation
- joint stiffness in the morning
- fatigue and moving slowly through life
- fluid retention and bloating
- depression, anxiety, and insomnia

Underfunctioning thyroid can put you at risk for many conditions such as poor lipid levels, elevated homocysteine, and elevated hsCRP, an inflammatory marker. Hypo- and hyperthyroidism are related to poor menstrual cycle symptoms and control. Hypothyroidism puts people at risk for congestive heart failure, low cardiac performance, poor growth, and poor remodeling after acute myocardial infarction (a heart attack). Suboptimal thyroid function can also be connected to low nitric oxide, an important compound in the body for circulation, vascular resistance (blood vessel health), and erection.

Optimizing thyroid function can offer great benefits, including promoting better control of blood sugar as well as reducing cardiovascular risk. Some of the many benefits are listed below. Sometimes the argument against optimizing the thyroid through thyroid replacement is that it can increase the risk for osteoporosis, but there are many studies supporting the fact that thyroid replacement, even when TSH is depressed, does not in fact increase osteoporosis risk.[52]

Benefits of optimizing the thyroid include:

- improved energy
- improved lipid profiles and decreased cardiovascular risk
- improved menstrual cycles
- improved cognitive ability and neuropsychiatric well-being
- reduced beta-amyloid plaque formation
- lowered hsCRP and homocysteine
- dilated coronary arteries
- improved blood pressure
- improved metabolic control (decreased metabolic syndrome issues, such as insulin resistance, and improved glycemic control)

Important Thyroid Hormones

It is important for you to understand the thyroid pathway of metabolism if you plan on going to your doctor and asking him or her to test your thyroid. I will warn you that what I am about to explain to you is not accepted by all doctors and can especially be rejected by many endocrinologists, but I assure you that the top doctors of the world know this information and use it to help their patients balance their hormones. I will discuss three important hormones. One hormone, the thyroid-stimulating hormone, or TSH, is secreted from the pituitary in the brain. Its job is exactly what its name says: it stimulates the thyroid to do its job, which is to make thyroid hormone. The two main thyroid hormones that the thyroid produces and secretes are referred to as T3, triiodothyronine, and T4, tetraiodothyronine. These molecules are named for how many iodine molecules they utilize—T3 uses three iodine molecules and T4 uses four. It is important to remember that while the body produces more T4, it is mostly an inactive compound, used only for storage purposes and conversion to T3 when it is needed for excess energy. The thyroid does secrete some T3, but in a much more limited quantity. T3 is your active thyroid hormone and the hormone that does most of the physiological work. It is also needed for fat loss. Your body works best when all these hormones are in balance, and they work based upon an intricate feedback loop that ensures they continue to communicate.

Impaired T4 to T3 Conversion

The body is reliant on an efficient conversion of T4 to T3 when needed by the tissues. There are various factors causing conversion from T4 to T3 to be less than ideal, and they are listed below.

- Endocrine
  » High cortisol
  » Low cortisol
  » Aging
  » GH deficiency
  » Glucose and insulin dysregulation
- Pharmaceutical
  » Glucocorticoids (cortisol and drugs that end in "one": cortisone, prednisone, prednisolone, dexamethasone, betamethasone, triamcinolone, fludrocortisone, aldosterone, etc.)
  » Beta blockers
  » Synthetic progestins
  » Amiodarone (antiarrhythmic drug)

In the ideal world, this feedback loop continues to communicate well and your TSH, T3, and T4 stay in optimal ranges. Research from childhood numbers reveal that free T3 levels are much higher than what is accepted as within normal limits for the average adult. Free T3 is the amount of T3 that is active and available in circulation. This is the true measure of how much activity your thyroid is able to produce for maintaining regular metabolism. Research into cardiovascular risk and parameters suggest that a free T3 level of less than 3.1 is predictive of increased death in cardiac patients, suggesting a strong connection between how well your "battery" is functioning and how healthy your heart and cardiovascular system are.[53]

Thyroid Testing

I suggest five initial blood tests for testing thyroid function. I always test TSH, free T3 (FT3), and free T4 (FT4), in addition to two tests to check autoimmune issues related to the thyroid. These tests are TPO, thyroid peroxidase, and anti-Tg, anti-thyroglobulin. This can give me an idea of whether or not a person suffers from Hashimoto's thyroiditis, a thyroid condition that is caused by an immune attack on the thyroid. If someone's TPO and anti-Tg are completely undetectable the first time I test him or her, I may not test them again for five years, knowing that they are likely to stay low. If they are elevated but the thyroid is still functioning well because TSH, FT3, and FT4 are all within normal limits, we may be catching the problem years before it will ever exhibit symptoms. This is important because lifestyle changes and improvements to the diet, such as removing gluten, can significantly reduce the autoimmune triggers and help to reduce TPO and anti-Tg.

A sixth important thyroid test can be run if we suspect that the patient's system has a high degree of toxicity, especially from heavy metals, or if the patient is under a lot of stress. Sometimes under these situations instead of the body converting T4 into T3, the body will convert T4 into a chemical similar to T3 but that malfunctions at receptor sites. This chemical is called reverse T3, or rT3. Detecting rT3 can help figure out a piece of the puzzle in many thyroid conditions.

Currently many doctors base thyroid function on one test alone, the TSH. However, testing TSH alone comes up short because it is a hormone that is secreted from the pituitary based upon feedback from T4 and T3. If the body has a lot of T4 but not enough T3, the pituitary will get the signal that everything is fine and the TSH level may look optimal. If doctors are only testing the TSH, they are not getting the whole picture. I can get a great idea of how the body is functioning and what other insults might be affecting the body by looking at the FT3 and FT4 levels. For example, if someone has high to normal FT3 and low FT4, they may be deficient in iodine. Contrastingly, if someone is normal in FT4 and low in FT3, they clearly have a conversion problem. And remember, the thyroid is like our battery and can have a significant effect on the body's ability to balance blood sugar levels and optimize hormone function in the pancreas and the liver to control blood sugar. Production of all enzymes will slow down if the thyroid isn't optimal.

Thyroid Medication

It is important to remember that not all thyroid medications are created equal. I like to think of the thyroid as the protector of all the other glands. Its function can affect many other systems like the adrenals and the ovaries; thus it plays a part in balancing the hormone system and menstrual cycle, as well as supporting the stress response. Most doctors, when prescribing thyroid medication, will use a version of T4 such as Levoxyl or Synthroid. When supplementing with T4 only, some imbalances may arise. For example, if someone is under stress and nutrient deficient, they may not be able to convert T4 to T3 readily, and therefore they can still have the symptoms of hypothyroidism because their T3 remains low. As mentioned above, if only checking TSH in a patient's blood work, all will look fine, but the patient will not feel any better.

Only prescribing T4 can also affect the ability of the thyroid to maintain healthy contraction of the heart if someone has difficulty converting T4 into T3. The heart only has receptors for T3; therefore it is dependent on the healthy conversion of T4 to T3. I prefer to use a thyroid medication such as Armour Thyroid or Nature-Throid because it is comprised of T4 and T3 and is better able to support the thyroid and the body in performing efficient daily metabolism. Westhroid is another T4/T3 blend that has even fewer additives. Westhroid was one of the first hypothyroid medications and it has never been recalled for inconsistencies. The thyroid hormones can also be compounded for someone who is interested in a vegetarian option. My experience with using compounded thyroid is that the absorption is poor; therefore, I need to use a much larger dose than I am used to.

Another way to accomplish balanced T4 and T3 when prescribing medication is with the use of a medicine in addtion to the regular T4 that many doctors are prescribing. For example, if someone is currently on levothyroxine and their FT4 levels are good but their FT3 levels are low, a prescription called Cytomel can be used. Cytomel is a synthetic version of T3. I don't often use this except in the rare cases of a vegetarian patient or someone who didn't do well on Armour or Nature-Throid.

Iodine Deficiency

Iodine deficiency refers to the deficiency of the trace element iodine. Iodine deficiency may be more common in our current society than you think. Iodine deficiency has been on the rise in the United States and other developed countries. In fact, iodine deficiency has increased fourfold in the past 40 years.[54] Part of this may be due to the poor iodine content of our foods and reduced sodium intake. We used to get enough iodine through eating iodized salt, but now the iodine quality in salt has declined, as has our natural consumption of salt. The health benefits of salt restriction have been well established in medical research, but we may be taking the word "restriction" a bit too far, into "elimination." Because salt can be connected with heart disease and elevated blood pressure and many processed foods are oversalted, we have gone on a quest to eliminate *all* salt from the diet, which may be to our detriment.

Iodine has a vital role in thyroid function. Iodine deficiency can increase the risk of developing fibrocystic breast disease, breast cancer, and hypothyroidism, may have a connection with chronic fatigue syndrome, and can promote goiter formation. A goiter is a large, sometimes painful swelling at the base of the neck and extending outwards. Large goiters can be seen and palpated, but small goiters can go unnoticed for a long time. Often, goiters are accompanied by thick necks.

In the 1920s, the United States recognized that goiters were as common as iodine deficiency, so we implemented a standard practice of consuming iodized salt. After this iodized salt introduction, the problem with goiter presentation decreased dramatically. But over time, we have begun to limit our salt consumption again, as well as consuming lower-quality salts that no longer contain iodine.

In addition to the increase in iodine deficiency, we have also witnessed environmental chemicals that interfere with the uptake and utilization of iodine. For example, a compound called perchlorate inhibits the thyroid from being able to absorb and utilize iodine. Perchlorate was originally designed for rocket fuel and explosives but is now found in ground water, soil, and even food items. I remember reading a study a while back about perchlorate being found in organic leafy greens that came from California. Interestingly, the perchlorate was nearly four times higher in the organic form of the greens compared to the non-organic. This gets a little scary. What I theorized from this was that the organic greens were extremely clean of toxins; therefore, they were able to absorb the perchlorate at a higher rate through the soil. So, we are obviously not ever completely free of being exposed to environmental toxins, no matter how safely we choose our vegetables at the store.

The take-away from this should be if you have a thyroid disorder or subclinical hypothyroid symptoms, fibrocystic breast disease, or persistent fatigue, you may, in fact, be iodine deficient. Various studies have been performed to deem safe doses iodine. Japanese women have an average iodine intake of between 5,280 mcg and 13,800 mcg with no side effects and many health benefits.[55]

Iodine Deficiency Testing

Iodine deficiency can be confirmed with an iodine loading test. Many labs do this test, and if you suspect you have iodine deficiency, you can request that your doctor perform this test. The test is performed by taking a large dose of iodine, equivalent to 50 mg, and then collecting your urine for 24 hours. Fifty milligrams is a very large dose, and I do not recommend you try to do this on your own or start taking 50 mg of iodine regularly. The test concept is simple. If you are iodine low, then you will keep most of the iodine and not urinate much out. If you have sufficient levels of iodine, you simply will excrete it. This is another reason that I am very comfortable with the use of iodine. If the body doesn't need it, it will excrete much of it out. For someone who has sufficient iodine and a well-balanced thyroid, however, taking iodine regularly may cause hyperthyroidism, which can cause hyperactivity of the thyroid. The symptoms of hyperthyroidism are explained below. Iodine use is usually best if combined with the use of selenium, an important antioxidant and an important nutrient for helping the conversion of T4 to T3.

Bromide Toxicity

Now that I have brought up the idea of using iodine to help support thyroid function and protect against breast cancer, I must briefly discuss bromide toxicity. Bromide is a compound found in our environment that competes with iodine for the same receptor sites in the body. If you are iodine low and have a lot of bromide bound up in your body/receptors, then when you start taking iodine, it can kick the bromide out. When this occurs, you can feel very sick, like you are detoxing. The reaction can be improved by drinking a lot of water, exercising, spending time in a hot sauna, and taking a lot of vitamin C and other antioxidants. If you continue using iodine, the symptoms will lessen. If the symptoms are too severe to handle, then you can reduce your iodine and increase the dose slowly over the course of weeks or months.

We don't see bromide toxicity symptoms unless we are using large doses of iodine (in the 12 mg and above range), which I don't suggest you do without guidance.

Hyperthyroidism

Hyperthyroidism is a more rare condition that occurs when the thyroid overproduces thyroid hormone. Hyperthyroidism symptoms can also be experienced if someone is taking too much thyroid hormone medication. Too much active thyroid in the body can cause unpleasant symptoms, such as anxiety, throat swelling, inability to sleep, fatigue, hair loss, brittle hair and nails, sudden weight loss, rapid heartbeat, sweating, chest pain, feeling like you are having a heart attack, and changes in bowel patterns. Many times, hypothyroidism can go undiagnosed, but hyperthyroidism is more likely to be diagnosed because the symptoms often are more acute. Usually, medical treatment of hyperthyroidism is more complex than treating hypothyroidism and can sometimes involve radiation treatment of the thyroid to stop its overproduction of hormone. Natural treatments can also be used to help the thyroid maintain its balance. Hyperthyroidism is often related to an autoimmune process in the body. TPO and anti-Tg should be included in the battery of tests used to determine the severity of hyperthyroidism. Although iodine may be used in some cases of hyperthyroidism under the supervision of a physician, I suggest all hyperthyroid patients avoid the use of iodine.

Adrenal Glands, the Adaptors

Another part of the hypothalamic axis is the adrenal glands. The adrenal glands were mentioned earlier; if you remember, they are responsible for balancing our stress response and helping to balance our blood sugar control. The adrenal glands are important in helping our body to adapt to its environment and are needed to maintain homeostasis of energy and stress chemicals. The adrenal glands secrete the important hormones cortisol and cortisone, estrogen, progesterone, other steroids, epinephrine, norepinephrine, and dopamine. Epinephrine is the familiar hormone that we refer to as adrenaline; it is secreted when we are revved up and excited about something. The adrenal glands must secrete hormones in consistent balance with other organs in the body. Too much of one hormone combined with too little of another can cause significant shifts in emotional balance and physical health. For example, too much norepinephrine combined with low dopamine can lead to high-anxiety states. Prolonged hormone imbalances can lead to increased oxidative stress, inflammation, and poor quality of life and sense of well-being. Prolonged oxidative stress from various means can constantly stress the adrenals, causing them to be continually stimulated. This can eventually cause adrenal burnout or fatigue. Many times when someone is fatigued, we assume that they must have a thyroid problem. Oftentimes, their thyroid is checked and it is fine, but they are still fatigued. There are a plethora of causes that need to be considered when assessing fatigue; therefore, fatigue is not pigeonholed to only poor adrenal gland function or burnout. But, adrenal fatigue should not be overlooked as an important phenomenon if someone has ongoing fatigue and all blood work panels appear normal.

The adrenal glands also secrete the steroid sex hormones estrogen, progesterone, and very small amounts of testosterone. Although the adrenal glands are not the main source for these hormones, during menopause and andropause states, the adrenals can be useful in picking up the slack left over by the inadequate secretion from the ovaries or testes. The adrenal glands are our glands of adaptation. They help us adapt to changes in our environment, especially when exposed to stressors such as deadlines, traffic, financial issues, and relationship stress, not to mention all the environmental stressors that we are exposed to on a daily basis. Unfortunately, the adrenal glands have done such a good job that we have packed on an abundance of stressful lifestyle routines. This is great for however many years our bodies are able to withstand the pressure. But not great when the adrenal glands are finally burnt out from the overwork and high demands on their function. Adrenal fatigue or burnout is common and can affect the secretion of many hormones important in controlling various processes in the body. Mainly, when the adrenal glands are burnt out, fatigue sets in, but many body processes under the tip of the iceberg are also affected.

Gonads, the Sex Glands

Due to an increase in emotional, mental, and physical stressors, people's hormones are decreasing significantly faster as they age. In some individuals, hormones that used to decrease in late life are starting to decline as early as the mid-20s. Depressed hormone levels in men and women put them at risk for serious chronic illness such as prostate cancer, breast cancer, and many cardiovascular diseases. Depressed hormones also cause a decreased sense of well-being and can affect quality of life and quality of relationships with others. I can make strong arguments for optimizing hormones for both men and women to improve blood sugar levels and quality of life. Here are merely some of the benefits of hormone optimization in both men and women:

- Longer life
- Reduced risk for chronic disease
- Reduced risk for cancers, such as prostate and breast
- Better energy, mood, zest for life

- Improved energy for making important lifestyle changes such as diet and exercise
- Better health to allow more individuals to contribute more to the workplace and society
- Healthier collective universe if many more people are happier and healthier

There is powerful research on the relationship between sex hormones and cardiovascular health, diabetes, and dementia. I will talk about a few basic hormones related to both male and female morbidity and mortality risks. The three I want to discuss are estrogen, progesterone, and testosterone. We think about estrogen and progesterone as female hormones but both are also found and are important in men.

Estrogen and Progesterone

Hormone balance is important. Any woman can tell you that she notices when her hormones are off. Imagine many of the diagnoses that women come to the doctor with that are related to an imbalance in hormones: menopausal symptoms, hot flashes, night sweats, PMS, postpartum depression, and infertility, just to name a few. But, there are many more conditions related to hormone balance, some obvious and some not. I think we are experiencing an epidemic of female conditions that are specifically related to low progesterone or, similarly, elevated estrogen.

Estrogen acts as a primer for testosterone and progesterone sexual effects. Having adequate estrogen levels as you age is important in prevention of Alzheimer's disease, autoimmune conditions, and osteoporosis. Estrogen is found in three main forms in the body: estriol, estradiol, and estrone.[56] Estriol, the main form of estrogen, controls over 400 functions in the body. It is neuroprotective, bone protective, and cardioprotective; can help prevent painful intercourse, vaginal atrophy, and incontinence; and reduces the risk of new-onset diabetes. Estriol offers breast cancer protection; decreases blood pressure, triglycerides, and total cholesterol; and helps to increase HDL, the "good" cholesterol. Estrogen is also important for men. Estrogen in men protects and maintains bone density and helps to prevent atherosclerosis. Additionally, low estrogen levels in men are associated with quicker mental decline. Caution, though: too much estrogen for men is definitely not desirable. Male estradiol levels shouldn't be below 20, but over 40 can be problematic.

Progesterone is an important hormone as it can impact mood, sleep, and overall sense of well-being. Even further, progesterone helps in maintaining level-headedness. Progesterone is also important for successful conception as it prepares the lining of the endometrium for implanting a fertilized egg. Each month when conception doesn't happen, the lining is shed. Progesterone helps balance blood sugar levels, boosts and regulates thyroid function, helps the breakdown of fat for use as energy, and helps to reduce swelling and inflammation. Progesterone is also extremely cardioprotective. Used along with either transdermal (topical use) or subcutaneous (implanted under the skin) estrogen, progesterone can help maintain blood pressure, lipid levels, and does not increase the risk of thrombosis or stroke. Micronized progesterone further reduces the incidence of new-onset diabetes when combined with transdermal estrogen, which suggests a role for progesterone in glucose regulation.[57]

Symptoms of low progesterone are:

- sugar cravings
- ovarian cysts
- irregular periods
- short luteal phase in menstrual cycle
- infertility
- endometriosis
- recurrent early miscarriage
- recurrent early delivery or having recurrent premature infants
- blood clots
- cold hands and feet
- decreased sex drive
- depression
- anxiety

- mood swings
- acne
- insomnia
- constant allergies
- fatigue
- slow metabolism

Estrogen Dominance

We just discussed the importance of estrogen, but many people have what we consider "estrogen dominance," which is a state within the body of elevated estrogen influence on tissues. Some people may have high estrogen levels that cause their estrogen dominance, but other individuals may have too little progesterone to balance out the amount of estrogen they have. Therefore, determining the true cause of estrogen dominance is an important first step when seeking to balance hormones.

Estrogen dominance can cause someone to have syptoms of low progesterone even if their progesterone levels are normal. When your estrogen is high, your body senses that your progesterone is low, even if it is not. Therefore, your body triggers symptoms of low progesterone because of the excess of estrogen.

Estrogen dominance, or excess estrogen, is becoming more common due to the increase in our environmental exposure to estrogen. One notable exposure is in some water supplies. Even in a closed environment, it has been shown that women's use of a form of topical estrogen in the home has led to elevated estrogen in family members as it is easily transferred from the hands of one person to another. Exposure has also come from accumulated estrogenlike compounds throughout our years of using plastics. These chemicals are called xenobiotic, and they fit similarly into estrogen receptors, making the body sense "extra estrogen" and sometimes even driving some metabolic processes within the body.

Finally, estrogen dominance is often seen associated with metabolic syndrome and obesity.

Humans are becoming larger, and with additional fat cells, we tend to accumulate more estrogen than we need. In an overweight individual, this excess estrogen can lead to low progesterone or low progesterone symptoms. My concern about the low progesterone/high estrogen problem is that we are seeing this imbalance lead to some dangerous conditions such as breast cancer, ovarian cancer, prostate cancer, and possibly uterine cancer. Excess estrogen, without the balance of progesterone, can be dangerous if left untreated.

I am not saying that everyone needs to take progesterone, but every woman should be aware of what her body is telling her. Early symptoms are the best way to determine estrogen to progesterone (E:P) balance. The good news is that an E:P imbalance can be discovered at a very young age, and it can be treated and prevented early. If, for instance, I see a fourteen-year-old girl having significant cramping, heavy bleeding, and PMS, my first line of treatment is to balance her E:P ratio so that she starts having a more comfortable cycle. What is important to her long-term health is keeping her hormones balanced when she is younger, so that she will have a better transition into fertility, will have healthier and better-balanced pregnancies, will transition into menopause more smoothly, and will have a better chance at preventing breast or ovarian cancer. This is a lot to think about for a fourteen-year-old, but I think of her future and feel grateful that I can play an early role in her longevity and well-being.

Stress Causes Low Progesterone

Progesterone may decrease when a person is under stress. You may know of someone who was under a great deal of stress and missed a few menstrual cycles. This occurs because the precursor hormone that is used to make progesterone and estrogen also has to make the stress hormone. When someone is under stress for any reason, stress always wins. Our bodies were designed that way evolutionarily for immediate survival. When we came across a tiger in the woods and needed to run from it, stress hormones prevailed to get us through that situation while turning off all our nonvital body processes such as menstrual cycles and digestion. Therefore, when we are under constant significant stress, it affects our hormone balance.

We have not yet evolved past this state of affairs; living under constant stress, as many people do, has certainly taken a toll on physiology and how all the organs of the body function together. The stress glands and the adrenals always win, and usually the organs that suffer are the ovaries and the thyroid. Therefore, when the adrenals are under stress, thyroid hormones and ovarian hormones, such as estrogen, progesterone, and testosterone, can be poorly regulated.

Taking progesterone is not always the best solution, depending on many factors, including age, whether one wants to get pregnant in the near future, family history of progesterone-sensitive breast cancers, and other key factors. Herbs and dietary habits can help with estrogen dominance, and reducing stress can help with stress-induced low progesterone.

Testosterone

Testosterone is one of my favorite hormones to discuss because people's awareness of it is very low compared to their awareness of estrogen and progesterone. Especially for women who are familiar with bioidentical hormone replacement, estrogen and progesterone are usually highlighted but testosterone is only minimally discussed. Testosterone plays a part in many important reactions in the body. There are many causes of testosterone loss such as natural menopause or andropause, childbirth, adrenal stress or burnout, endometriosis, depression, chronic use of birth control pills, HMG-CoA reductase inhibitors (pharmaceutical medications used to treat elevated cholesterol levels), chemotherapy, and aging, just to name a few. Interestingly, after 10 years of oral birth control use, libido drops significantly, most likely due to lowered testosterone levels. Fatigue is one of the most common symptoms expressed by my patients. Most of my patients want more energy and to feel like they felt when they were younger. As adrenal gland function is often overlooked in the differential diagnosis of fatigue, so low testosterone is also overlooked. Low testosterone, sometimes occurring very early in young men and women, can promote a significant and confounding fatigue. If doctors don't know to look into low testosterone levels in men and women, the etiology may be missed for years.

Sometimes simply supporting the adrenal glands, reducing stress, and using supportive supplements can help improve testosterone levels in younger men and women. As people age, it is more difficult to improve testosterone levels without the use of supplemental testosterone.

Symptoms associated with low testosterone are:

- tendency toward increased abdominal fat
- low libido
- less energy and tiring from physical activity
- loss of muscle tone
- changes in cognition and/or memory loss
- anxiety
- migraines (women)
- breasts getting fatty (men)
- erectile dysfunction (men)
- hot flashes and sweats (men)
- low self-esteem (more in men)

In four major studies, testosterone deficiency was linked to an increased risk of all-cause mortality. Low testosterone has been connected to elevated fasting glucose and elevated two-hour postprandial glucose levels. Low testosterone is also connected to poor lipid profiles such as elevated triglycerides, total cholesterol, and elevated LDL cholesterol. ApoA1 lipoprotein elevations, hypertension, and high blood pressure have been linked to testosterone deficiency. Additionally, low testosterone puts people at risk of developing type 2 diabetes mellitus and metabolic syndrome.

Testosterone is very important in bone density, maybe even more so than estrogen and calcium. We get so pigeonholed into thinking the same things over and over again, and when something is presented to us for years, it becomes ingrained in our memories and our beliefs. So, what have we been taught? At least for women, we have been taught that you should drink your milk, get in the sun for vitamin D levels, take calcium, and get on some bioidentical estrogen to preserve bone health, but low testosterone in both men and women is connected to increased risk for fracture.

Specifically, a study presented in the *Journal of Clinical Endocrinology Metabolism* in 2010 showed that low testosterone in men is related to a significantly increased risk for osteoporosis, heart disease, diabetes type 2, obesity, metabolic syndrome, and overall increased inflammation.[58]

There was a 10-year prospective study published on this topic by the National Institutes of Health which studied over 11,000 men 40 to 79 years old. This study found that those with high endogenous testosterone had low mortality from cardiovascular disease and cancer. Men in this study who had testosterone in the 1,000 range had a 57 percent decreased chance of dying due to all causes.[59] Men with testosterone lower than 900 had an increased risk for developing Alzheimer's disease. High testosterone in men is not associated with increased risk for prostate cancer. This is the main concern that I get from patients if we discuss testosterone use. Interestingly, elevated levels of estrone are related to increased risk for prostate cancer. This means that estrogen levels are more closely linked to prostate cancer than levels of testosterone.

Testosterone is also important for quality of life. Having low testosterone can make someone feel very fatigued, have a lower sense of self-esteem, experience low libido, and have less desire for the day-to-day activities in life. Decreases in testosterone can begin early in life and may not only be associated with natural aging. Because I am seeing low testosterone in 30-year-olds and even some 20-year-olds, there is something occurring in our environments that is increasing the probability of deficiency.

Pineal Gland, the Balancer

The pineal gland is a pinecone-shaped gland located near the center of the brain. Melatonin is an important hormone secreted by the pineal gland. One of its main jobs is to facilitate sleep, but it is a much more significant hormone than we once understood. Melatonin is found in all organisms, even bacteria, and it is always 10–15 times higher at night. It has significant antioxidant properties, scavenges free radicals, and thus can play a part in the prevention of chronic illness. Melatonin is important in immune modulation and inflammation control. It is protective for the arteries and can prevent blood pressure problems. One of the main reasons I have included it in my list of important hormones is because it plays a positive role in regulating insulin.[60] Additionally, a study published in the *Journal of the American Medical Association* in 2013 reported that problems with the melatonin receptor resulted in increased insulin resistance and type 2 diabetes. The study also found that low levels of melatonin at night were associated with increased insulin resistance.[61] If you connect this with those who are not sleeping well or not going to bed early enough, their problem may be that they just aren't sleeping enough hours to secrete enough melatonin to balance their insulin response. Another great point for making sure you get adequate sleep nightly.

Vitamin D, the Immune Modulator

Vitamin D has been misnamed because the name suggests that it is a vitamin or nutrient. What many people don't understand is that vitamin D is actually an extremely important hormone needed for balance and stimulation of the immune system. One way vitamin D is highlighted in the immune system is by being involved in the suppression of inflammatory cytokines. If you remember from our inflammation description, cytokines are chemical signalers that trigger inflammatory or anti-inflammatory responses. Vitamin D is important in helping calcium lay down bone matrix, leading to healthy bone density. As people age, bone deterioration occurs as a slow degradation due to multiple factors. Peak bone mass in women occurs anywhere from age 20 to 44 and decreases from then on.[62] This age range is wide because of various factors including cigarette smoking, diet, exercise, family history, hormone balance, and so on. Vitamin D works alongside vitamin K2 and vitamin A to help maintain healthy bones.

All cells have receptors for 1,25-dihydroxyvitamin D, also called calcitriol, the active form of vitamin D.

Vitamin D deficiency can increase overall disease risk. For example, having less than 15 ng/ml of 25-hydroxyvitamin D, the inactive form of vitamin D, is related to a two-and-a-half-fold increased risk for acute myocardial infarction and acute heart attack.[63] Low vitamin D increases infectious disease risk. Low vitamin D is also linked to double the rate of dementia, Alzheimer's, and stroke. Interestingly, diabetes mellitus type 1 incidence increases the further away from the equator the person lives. The conclusion from this is that the further away you move from the equator, the less close you are to the sun and the lower your vitamin D levels. Low neonatal vitamin D is also associated with increased risk for diabetes mellitus type 1.

Vitamin D deficiency is appearing in people who have chronic inflammatory disorders. 25-hydroxyvitamin D has been identified as a secosteroid. Secosteroids act to depress inflammation, which is why we see low vitamin D levels in many people who are plagued with inflammatory disorders.

Vitamin D can act as an aromatase inhibitor, especially in breast cancer. The enzyme aromatase converts testosterone into estrogen, so this can be important in breast cancer treatment and prevention. In many cases of breast cancer, the main goal is to keep estrogen levels low because breast cancer growth can increase in the presence of estrogen. Using pharmaceutical aromatase inhibitors presents many complications and side effects; therefore, if optimizing a patient's vitamin D levels can offer even mild aromatase inhibition, it is worthwhile to do so.

The vitamin D receptor, VDR, affects the transcription of multiple genes and therefore impacts processes ranging from calcium metabolism to immune modulation, and most likely is involved in processes beyond our current understanding. During exposure to infection, the body will convert inactive 25-hydroxyvitamin D to active 1, 25-dihydroxyvitamin D. As 1,25-dihydroxyvitamin D increases in the body, it activates the VDR and can stimulate various processes within the body. The body increases and decreases the production of 1,25-dihydroxyvitamin D to control the innate immune response. If a bacterial insult within the body is sustained, it can cause long-term effects on the balance of inactive versus active forms of vitamin D.

CHAPTER 8

Other Health Risks: Are You at Risk for Chronic Inflammation, Heart Disease, Cancer, or Diabetes?

There are a number of ways you can better understand your risk for heart disease, cancer, diabetes, and other chronic illnesses. First, you can take a look at your family history. You may not get everything your previous family members have suffered, but you may have increased risk for the ailments they acquired. For example, if you have family members with diabetes, you are more likely to acquire the disease as well. It is difficult to determine whether the increased risk among family members is through the learned environment of eating and lifestyle habits or through genetics. My guess is that it is a little bit of both. If a parent has type 2 diabetes, the risk of their child getting diabetes is one in seven if the parent was diagnosed before age 50 and one in 13 if the diagnosis was after age 50.[64] Obesity is another disease that has mixed genetic and environmental influences. An article published in *Child and Adolescent Psychiatric Clinics of North America* revealed that at least 50 percent of causative factors for child-hood obesity were genetic in nature, as they have been able to link obesity to the first polygenes involved in body weight regulation. [65]Cardiovascular disease has also been linked to genetic inheritance as well as poor diet and lifestyle choices.

You are most likely familiar with the genetic risks for cancer. For example, the BRCA gene is being tested heavily in women who have a family history of breast cancer to determine if they have the gene that will increase their own risk for cancer. There are various other examples of genes that are connected with cancer, but you need to also remember that some woman who have the gene still don't get cancer and vice versa. This just goes to show you how other influences can be just as important as genetic ones, and if you can put your genes in the healthiest environment possible, you have the ability to influence which genes are turned on and which are turned off.

The moral of the story is that genes are not everything, and that sometimes looking deeper into the body through regular blood work can give us a better clue of how patients are doing at any given moment in time. Regular blood tests let us assess a patient's progression of disease or improvement. If one of my patients is using a medication, herb, or supplement of any kind, I will expect to see a certain response in the patient. If I don't see it and my patient feels worse, I will reevaluate. Additionally, I like to use sense of well-being as a way to assess my patients. If a patient's sense of well-being worsens based on something we are doing, we will stop and reevaluate what is going on. Still, blood tests are not the be-all and end-all. You must put everything together, including all aspects of a person's being, in order to bring about wellness.

Following are some important cardiovascular disease tests. DON'T SKIP THIS SECTION. I tell you this because currently cardiovascular disease kills more people in the world than any other illness. And on top of that, it still remains the number-one killer in both women and men. Having some or all of these blood tests done may help you better evaluate your risks.

Important Testing to Evaluate Your Risks

Sometimes it is clear from a person's genetic history that he or she is at risk for developing an illness that is related to inflammation. Obesity, heart disease, diabetes, and many other inflammation-related conditions run in families. Take a good look at your elders' and siblings' health history and decide for yourself if you may be at risk. I would say that most individuals are at risk for inheriting some form of an inflammatory condition. Sometimes we inherit the probability through genetics, but we can also inherit it through learned behaviors around food, exercise, and our reaction to stress. Growing up in a household with family members who are sedentary and who frequently indulge in fast food almost guarantees that you'll need to exert yourself to adopt new habits. It is no longer enough to simply measure your total cholesterol and your blood pressure.

Here are a few tests that can help you understand your risks better:

- erythrocyte sedimentation rate (ESR)
- high-sensitivity C-reactive protein (hsCRP)
- fibrinogen
- lipoprotein-associated phospholipase A2 (Lp-PLA2)
- myeloperoxidase (MPO)
- fasting glucose levels
- hemoglobin A1c (HbA1c)
- fasting and postprandial insulin levels
- lipid panel
- apolipoprotein B (apo B)
- apolipoprotein A1 (apo A1)
- lipoprotein a (Lp(a))
- homocysteine
- B-type natriuretic peptide (BNP)

Erythrocyte Sedimentation Rate (ESR)

Sed rate, or erythrocyte sedimentation rate (ESR), can be tested at a doctor's office to determine how much inflammation is present in one's system. This figure is not a stand-alone diagnostic tool, but along with other blood work and a complete history and physical, it can be extremely helpful in diagnosing and treating a patient. When a patient's blood is placed in a tall, thin tube, red blood cells (erythrocytes) gradually settle to the bottom. Inflammation can cause the cells to clump together. Because clumps of cells are denser than individual cells, they settle to the bottom more quickly. The sed rate test measures the distance red blood cells fall in a test tube in one hour. The farther the red blood cells have descended, the greater the inflammatory response of the patient's immune system. ESR is often elevated in individuals suffering from arthritis or autoimmune disease. ESR may be more helpful in monitoring a patient's response to treatment than in determining a diagnosis.

There are many causes for an increase in ESR, and ESR is not regularly monitored in cardiac or diabetic patients. I like to use it as a screening tool initially so I can gather as much information about my patient's internal environment as possible. If elevated, it can alert me to an acute process of inflammation that needs to be addressed. Oftentimes, I see ESR elevated in rheumatoid and other forms of arthritis, inflammatory bowel disease, acute infection, bone infections, and various other conditions. An extreme elevation of the ESR is strongly associated with serious underlying disease, most often infection, collagen vascular disease, or metastatic malignancy. If I see an elevated ESR, I initiate an anti-inflammatory protocol, better diet, and exercise, and then I will recheck it after an interval of time to see if it is improving. If it hasn't moved or increased but is still concerningly elevated, I will then conduct further tests to determine the cause of the elevation.

High-Sensitivity C-Reactive Protein (hsCRP)

Often, ESR is coupled with other tests. High-sensitivity C-reactive protein, or hsCRP, is another major test that reveals chronic inflammation. The level of hsCRP, a protein found in the blood, rises in response to inflammation. Studies have shown that persistent low-grade inflammation is connected to atherosclerosis, the narrowing of blood vessels as a result of buildup of cholesterol and other lipids. It's important to note that levels of hsCRP increase and decrease due to various health issues, so one cannot assume that if it is elevated it is always related to the cardiovascular system. For example, hsCRP may be elevated due to an autoimmune-related disease or arthritis. Even if the hsCRP is elevated due to a noncardiovascular cause the elevated hsCRP can increase cardiovascular disease risk. Some of the main reasons hsCRP could be elevated include, but are not limited to, acute or chronic infection, inflammatory bowel disease, autoimmune diseases such as rheumatoid arthritis, cardiovascular disease, cancer, poor diet, sedentary lifestyle, and exposure to environmental irritants.

hsCRP can decrease from the use of NSAIDs, as well as statin drugs used to lower cholesterol. It may be elevated in women taking oral estrogen in any form, including estradiol.

The school of thought on using hsCRP to determine or monitor cardiovascular risk is still largely conflicted among medical experts and physicians. I use it first as an initial screening tool in my patients and then if elevated, I will use it to help me understand if their inflammation levels are improving or worsening over time. It helps me better evaluate whether the treatments we are using are effective or need to be altered to better suit the patient. Additionally, I will periodically monitor hsCRP in my cancer survivors because if it is low and then spikes, it can give me an idea that there might be something going on internally, and then we can catch cancer recurrence much quicker than we would have if we hadn't done the test.

The American Heart Association and US Centers for Disease Control and Prevention have defined risk groups as follows:

- Low risk: less than 1.0 mg/L
- Average risk: 1.0 to 3.0 mg/L
- High risk: above 3.0 mg/L

Fibrinogen

Fibrinogen is a clotting protein and is associated with the inflammatory cascade. Fibrinogen may be elevated during acute and chronic inflammation. Excess fibrinogen can help gauge elevated clotting risk, risk of plaque, and risk of stroke. Elevated fibrinogen is proportionally risky for cardiovascular disease. For example, the higher your fibrinogen, the higher your risk for cardiovascular disease. Therefore, if someone has elevated fibrinogen and already has heart disease, working toward decreasing inflammation, decreasing oxidative stress, and improving fibrinogen levels may result in improved cardiovascular risk.

Lipoprotein-Associated Phospholipase A2 (Lp-PLA2)

Lipoprotein-associated phospholipase A_2 (Lp-PLA$_2$) is another marker of inflammation. It is an enzyme that is secreted by macrophages and monocytes, cells of the immune system. Lp-PLA$_2$ is being looked at in cardiovascular disease because higher levels of Lp-PLA$_2$ are associated with increased risk for atherosclerosis. Combine this with elevated hsCRP levels and stroke risk increases significantly.

Myeloperoxidase (MPO)

Myeloperoxidase (MPO) is another enzyme made by immune cells. MPO is made specifically by immune cells that are located in the blood vessel walls. So we know when it is elevated that something is going on specifically in the blood vessels. Extremely elevated MPO, such as over 630, is associated with an increased risk for major cardiac events, even more so if hsCRP is elevated as well. Simultaneous elevated levels of MPO, hsCRP, and Lp-PLA$_2$ are associated with markedly increased risk of a major cardiac event within the next six months.

Fasting Glucose

Fasting glucose can be immediately tested at home with a glucometer, a machine that uses a drop of blood to determine how much blood sugar is detected. It can also be tested at a physician's office, hospital, or lab with results that will come back within 24 hours. For someone who doesn't have diabetes, it is not warranted to have a glucometer at home; therefore, the testing will usually be performed by a physician's order. Most likely, if you are seeing a primary care doctor, this will be included with your yearly blood tests. To prepare for a fasting glucose level, you need to not eat anything for 12 hours before the test. Drinking water is allowed, but no other beverages.

Often these tests are performed in the morning so that you can easily fast through the night for the test.

Fasting glucose levels can give us an idea of how the body is managing the balance between how much sugar is in the blood-stream and how much is allowed to pass into the cells in the tissues. Fasting glucose is best under 100 mg/dl and the body will strive for this number, even if it means increasing insulin levels. It is extremely important to be on top of this issue as soon as you see it arise. If you can catch elevated blood glucose or even elevated insulin early, you can implement some significant diet and lifestyle changes that can reverse the disease process. Even if your blood glucose is not above 100, if you start to compare your previous lab tests and you see your number increasing from 80 to 99 throughout the years, you may be starting to have glucose regulation problems. In this case, you may want to have your insulin levels tested.

As you can imagine, the longer the blood glucose problem has been present and the higher the glucose and insulin numbers, the slower the reversal and the longer it takes to get the glucose back to normal. I suggest that the quest for maintaining balanced glucose levels be a lifelong endeavor. That means that if you are struggling with glucose problems, then make it your lifelong effort to continue improving and working on your diet and lifestyle habits. It is worth it to change now so that your future health is good. Spending time with your grandchildren and great-grandchildren, and maintaining a healthy mental and emotional function should motivate you to con-tinue on your quest for wellness.

Hemoglobin A1c (HbA1c)

Glycated hemoglobin is one of my favorite tests. It can give us an idea of what your blood sugar average has been over the three months prior to the test. It is not an average of fasting glucose levels, rather an average of random glucose levels. This test is especially useful if someone has always had normal glucose but then has a test that reveals elevated glucose. Have they just been eating poorly for the two weeks before, or are they having significant glucose control issues? If you remember the earlier discussion of glycated hemoglobin in relationship to AGEs, you'll recall that if hemoglobin A1c is elevated, the risk for oxidative damage to the tissues, including blood vessels, is elevated as well. Hemoglobin A1c levels rise when there is a lot of sugar in the blood that bonds with hemoglobin molecules. A hemoglobin A1c level should be checked every three months in someone with diabetes or prediabetes to determine if the treatment plan, diet, and lifestyle changes are effective.

The normal range for hemoglobin A1c for people without diabetes is between 4.5 percent and 5.6 percent, estimating average nonfasting glucose to be between 83 and 114. Hemoglobin A1c levels between 5.7 percent and 6.4 percent indicate increased risk of diabetes, and levels of 6.5 percent or higher indicate diabetes. I have included a chart below so that you are able to view the relationship between glucose levels and hemoglobin A1c. I included quite high levels because it is not uncommon to find a hemoglobin A1c of, say, 12.5 percent in someone who is not controlling their blood sugar levels well.

Hemoglobin A1c	Average Glucose Level
4 *hypoglycemia	68
4.5 *normal glucose levels	83
5	97
5.5	111
5.6	114
5.7 *increased diabetes risk	117
6	126
6.4	137
6.5 *diabetes diagnosis	140
7	154
7.5	169
8	183
8.5	197
9	215

9.5	226
10	240
10.5	255
11	269
11.5	283
12	298
12.5	312
13	326
13.5	341
14 +	Scary!

Fasting and Postprandial Insulin Levels

Another test that can help us understand how the body is coping with blood sugar balance is fasting and sometimes after-eating insulin levels. Interestingly, because the body is so good at maintaining homeostasis, the blood glucose may be normal for many years while a diabetes disease process is building. To help you understand this more, when the body is stressed with elevated glucose levels, it may begin to produce more insulin to allow the passage of blood sugar out of the bloodstream and into the tissues. Therefore, when you are checked, your blood sugar may look normal, but your insulin may be really high in order to facilitate this delicate balance. The very first sign we may see if someone is struggling with their blood sugar control may be normal glucose with elevated insulin. If we don't check the insulin levels, then this increased insulin can go unnoticed for many years, leading eventually to insulin resistance and subsequent pancreatic burnout, which I discussed in chapter 4.

Insulin levels can be anywhere from three or four to in the teens or twenties. I believe the optimal level of insulin lies in the 6-10 range. I understand this is a tight range, but anything outside of it can show insulin dysregulation, even if fasting blood glucose levels are within normal limits. The good news for teenagers who are eating a lot of sugar and have elevated insulin levels is that it is pretty easy to stop consuming sugar and have insulin levels come back down to normal levels. But the longer your insulin is out of balance, the more you increase your potential of insulin resistance, metabolic syndrome, and eventually diabetes. The older you are, the harder it is to regulate insulin levels; therefore, sometimes a very strict and aggressive plan is needed for older patients to bring insulin back into balance.

Lipid Panel

Lipid panels give us little information on true cardiovascular risk. The main components of a lipid panel are total cholesterol, LDL cholesterol, HDL cholesterol, and triglycerides. Other components of a lipid panel may include very-low-density lipoprotein (VLDL) cholesterol level.

Cholesterol, which is an essential substance in the body, is located in cell membranes and is a precursor to many of the important steroid hormones mentioned earlier. Although cholesterol is important in the body, elevated plasma levels may be associated with the development of atherosclerotic plaque formation within blood vessels. Myocardial infarction, or heart attack, can be the end result of significant atherosclerotic plaque. Cholesterol is only one component of lipoproteins, so merely testing total plasma cholesterol is no longer adequate in determining someone's cardiovascular risk.

Elevated low-density lipoprotein (LDL) cholesterol has been identified in various studies as possibly increasing the risk of cardiovascular disease in both men and women. High-density lipoprotein (HDL) cholesterol is believed to be the protective cholesterol, or "good" cholesterol. While in part this is true, HDL is actually a complex group of molecules. Some of the HDL cholesterol acts appropriately as large garbage trucks, cleansing the blood vessels of debris and excess waste, thereby acting protectively to the arteries and other blood vessels. There are a few types of HDL cholesterol molecules, though, that are rather small, and instead of doing a good job of cleansing the artery, their small size can increase the risk of causing microdamage to the blood vessel or getting lodged into an already forming plaque. Therefore, it isn't correct to assume that if your HDL cholesterol levels are high, they are appropriately protective. Again, LDL is considered the "bad" cholesterol, but not all of its processes are bad or harmful. In fact, the body needs LDL. In large quantities, LDL has the potential to harm arteries; therefore, we want to keep it at a balanced level in the body.

Apolipoprotein B (Apo B)

Apolipoprotein B, Apo B, is a component of many lipoproteins that are involved in atherosclerosis and cardiovascular disease. Apo B is produced in the liver and intestines, and it provides structure to the triglyceride molecule. A measure of Apo B is a direct measure of how many atherogenic particles are in circulation. In other words, the level of Apo B is directly related to how much risk someone has for developing atherosclerosis. Testing for levels of apolipoprotein B may reveal more about cardiac health than simply measuring LDL. Apo B is a stronger predictor of cardiovascular disease than LDL cholesterol.

Apolipoprotein A1 (Apo A1)

Apo A1 is a protein that is also made in the liver and intestine. It is a component of the HDL cholesterol; therefore, lower levels are associated with increased cardiovascular disease.

Lipoprotein A (Lp(a))

Lipoprotein A is a lipoprotein that is genetically determined. Because levels don't fluctuate quickly, treatments have not been targeted at lowering lipoprotein A. Elevated levels of lipoprotein A are associated with increased risks for atherosclerosis, coronary heart disease, and stroke. When elevated levels are found, the information can be used to formulate a more aggressive treatment plan for cardiovascular disease prevention. Lipoprotein A isn't a routine cardiac test but can be used to better assess future cardiovascular risk.

Homocysteine

Homocysteine is used by the body for repair. It helps to build and maintain tissue and is important in the manufacture of proteins. Elevated levels may mean your body is having to do repair work. Levels over 15 μmol/L have a strong relationship with cardiovascular disease and dementia. Any level over 10 µmol/L should be treated.

Brain Natriuretic Peptide (BNP)

Brain natriuretic peptide, also called B-type natriuretic peptide (BNP), is a neurohormone protein produced by the heart and blood vessels that helps the body eliminate fluids, relaxes blood vessels, and funnels sodium into the urine. It may be present in high levels if the heart is under stress or damaged. Elevated levels may identify dysfunction of the left ventricle of the heart. This is most likely associated with congestive heart failure. In cardiac patients, higher levels of BNP are associated with higher risk of morbidity and mortality.

Red Flags

As you can see, many of these markers tell us when there are deeper issues going on. This goes back to the unique ability of the body to do what is needed to survive. The body doesn't increase a substance like homocysteine or cholesterol to kill you. It does so because a repair job is needed somewhere. Think of these blood test markers in your blood work as red flags. "Oops, my cholesterol is up; I had better change something to improve it." Or, "Looks like my homocysteine is elevated; that means my body must be working on something. I should do all that I can to remove excess stress on the body to allow it to heal, and I should take action to support the cardiovascular system in general."

Cholesterol Changes Are Not Always Diet Related

Cholesterol can be accumulated two ways: through the diet (exogenously) and made by the liver (endogenously). Many people think that the main problem with elevated cholesterol levels is diet, but many people can have elevated cholesterol despite their diet. If someone eats fast food often, eats a lot of sugar, and lives sedentarily, then we would expect them to have elevated triglycerides in addition to high cholesterol, especially LDL cholesterol. However, many people have changed their diets and don't consume a diet high in cholesterol and unhealthy fats, but they continue to have elevated cholesterol.

Cholesterol is made in the liver for various purposes. For one, it is a precursor to all steroid hormones, including estrogen, progesterone, testosterone, and the important stress hormone cortisol. A body going through a lot of stress or hormone changes will elevate cholesterol as a way to increase these hormones. It is a very protective molecule (when not present in excess); therefore, the body will increase cholesterol when under physical stress (such as during elevated chronic inflammation). Cholesterol is a fat molecule and does a good job of absorbing toxicity; therefore, many people with internal health problems will have elevated cholesterol. Cholesterol is also very important in brain function and is an important part of the cell membrane.

Is Your Cholesterol Elevated Because of Your Diet?

Here is an easy way to examine and evaluate your blood work to determine if diet is the true cause of your elevated cholesterol. If you look at your numbers and your HDL is low (under 40), your LDL is high (over 125), and your total cholesterol is over 200, you are not looking so good. Now look at your triglycerides. This is the true answer. If your TGs are in the 250s or higher, then you can significantly change your cholesterol through dietary changes. If you have been doing everything you can to change your cholesterol through diet and your triglycerides are 45, then we know 100 percent that your elevated cholesterol has nothing to do with your diet. This doesn't mean that you should eat whatever you want, but it does mean that you can't just sit there with elevated cholesterol continuing to think that if you just do a little bit better with your diet, then your cholesterol will decrease. Please consult a naturopathic physician for further advice on decreasing your cholesterol, or contact your regular physician to take action focused on improving your cholesterol levels.

The National Institute of Nutrition recommends that every individual consume at least 300 grams of vegetables (50 g of green leafy vegetable, 200 g of other vegetables, and 50 g of root vegetables) and 100 grams of fruit daily. I would say that if we are trying to tightly control blood sugar, make sure those vegetables and fruits are on your okay-to-eat list.

Statin Drugs—Should We Use Them?

Statin drugs are the most commonly used drugs in America. Not surprisingly, doctors and other health professionals have us all running scared from elevated cholesterol levels. Though elevated cholesterol levels aren't something to laugh about, they are certainly not a death sentence. Many factors lead to advanced heart disease and heart attack. Cholesterol is only one of the major risk factors for cardiac events.

Pharmaceutical medications aimed at lowering cholesterol do only that: lower cholesterol. Yes, they may reduce the risk of heart attack, but they are not changing the picture or working to reverse the disease process that is occurring. In fact, they may be taking cholesterol away from important places that need it, like the brain. Cholesterol is a good transporter; therefore, if the body has high toxicity or inflammation, often cholesterol levels will increase. The solution to pollution is dilution. Cholesterol is a waxy, fatlike substance that tends to cause a diluting effect by swallowing the "bad" chemicals in the body. If the body is increasing cholesterol to act as protection, then it will be unlikely to give that cholesterol up. A cholesterol-lowering drug targets not only the cholesterol in the bloodstream but may also target the cholesterol that is used for other mechanisms such as hormone manufacture or nervous system support. Your body will be much more willing to let these mechanisms go because it will always prioritize survival. We know this by reviewing what occurs under stress. During an extremely stressful situation, the body will completely shut off digestion and healing because it is more concerned about immediate survival. Let me repeat this: the body will do anything to survive. All symptoms we see are the result of the body's attempt to stay alive.

A study published in 2012 in the *Archives of Internal Medicine* involving research from a significant number of women in the Women's Health Initiative Trial revealed a shocking 48 percent increased risk of developing diabetes among those women taking statin drugs.[66] The two main side effects associated with the use of cholesterol medication are memory loss and muscle weakness or fatigue. To recap, taking a drug will only stop your body from making the cholesterol; it will not stop the body's problem that triggered the cholesterol production in the first place. Changing the body's internal environment so that it no longer feels it necessary to make more cholesterol is the true answer.

Another significant side effect from taking statin drugs is low libido; low testosterone levels have been found among many statin drug users. The simple explanation to this is that testosterone and other important hormones have the cholesterol molecule as their main backbone, and if cholesterol levels are decreased in the body then hormones may decrease as well. In 2012, the FDA implemented safety label changes to statin medications to include more risks and warnings relating to issues such as liver complications, memory loss and confusion, unusual fatigue, elevated blood sugar levels, and others. [67]

Diabetes and Lipids and Increased Risk for Alzheimer's Disease

The incidence of Alzheimer's is increasing. Currently it is the sixth leading cause of death in the United States. It is not too early to start prevention of Alzheimer's disease, and it is not too late to begin a healthy diet once you have the early signs of Alzheimer's disease or dementia. Changing your diet now can drastically change your future. Copious research suggests a few direct connections between diet and Alzheimer's. For example, according to a study performed at Mount Sinai School of Medicine in New York City, high-protein diets led to "shrinking" of the brain in mice.[68] We have already observed in recent studies that patients with severe Alzheimer's can lose up to 20 percent of their brain mass. So I caution my patients about over-consumption of protein, especially since many of the new diet fads push higher protein intake. Although I do think protein is important and I do help my patients figure out ways of eating protein healthily, I stress the importance of whole vegetable and fruit intake above all other foods, including grains.

There is good news, though! We have the power to choose what we eat. Not all protein types lead to Alzheimer's and dementia. Maybe we aren't eating the right kinds of protein. Many studies have reported that increased omega-3 fatty acid intake is linked to lower incidence of Alzheimer's and dementia.[69] The moral of the story is: Don't increase your protein intake by eating a lot of hamburgers, but make sure you are eating more cold-water fish such as salmon.

What I am going to say next is going to seem like a "no brainer" to some of you, but maybe, just maybe, we know this information but don't live by it. Studies suggest that diets high in whole vegetables, fruits, and healthy fats reduce the risk of Alzheimer's disease and dementia, and diets high in saturated fats and sugary foods increase the risk of Alzheimer's disease and dementia. Studies support the notion that foods with a high glycemic index can directly lead to dementia. Studies have shown that diets high in flavonoid-rich berries delay memory decline and can play a part in delaying cognitive aging. Following an anti-inflammatory diet while paying attention to consuming low–glycemic index foods is a way to decrease your risk. In fact, eating an anti-inflammatory diet while consuming mostly low–glycemic index foods will help you reduce the risk of most of the leading causes of death in the United States. We already understand that eight of the top 10 leading causes of death are directly related to increased inflammation.

Statin Drugs and Alzheimer's

One other clinical pearl that I would like to share with you is the effect of statin drugs on Alzheimer's disease. I have seen multiple patients who come in with Alzheimer's disease that have been on statin drugs for many years. It is my impression that statin drugs that reduce cholesterol too much and for too long lead to reduction of cholesterol in the brain, and consequently lead to increased risk for dementia. Various studies confirm that statins continue to fail at preventing Alzheimer's disease, but I haven't seen one study yet on the potential link between statin use and the increased incidence of Alzheimer's. In fact, in one study published online in 2008 from the journal *Neurology*, researchers reported they were surprised that statin drugs did not reduce stroke or cerebral infarction pathology!

Even the Framingham heart study, which has been a popular cardiovascular-risk study for the past 50 years, has ongoing research into cholesterol levels and cognitive ability associations. According to the study's published report in 2005, cholesterol levels are highly associated with measures of verbal fluency, attention and concentration, abstract reasoning, and overall ability to perform well on the tests provided.[70] The relationship they found was proportional, meaning the higher cholesterol levels were, the higher the participants scored on their tests and the participants with lower cholesterol levels ("desirable" levels according to cardiovascular standards), did more poorly on their tests of verbal fluency, attention and concentration, abstract reasoning, and overall ability to execute the test. Again, supporting the fact that cholesterol has a protective effect on the brain and its overall functioning. It's important to remember that the brain contains about 25 percent of the cholesterol in the body, even though the brain itself is only a mere percentage of the body. Additionally cholesterol can represent almost 50 percent of the cell membrane of every cell in the body. By no means does cholesterol take a back seat, and we shouldn't use strong drugs to make it take one or the effects will be detrimental to health.

Current Lifestyle and Dietary Habits Age Us and Lead to Chronic Illness

This is a concept that you should understand well at this point in your reading of this material. The current dietary and lifestyle choices made by so many in our society—including consuming foods of poor nutrient quality (e.g., processed foods, junk foods, sweetened drinks, candy, pastries, cakes), engaging in sedentary habits and negative thinking, and succumbing to excess stress—send us to the grave. Frankly put, our diets, lack of exercise, and the amount of stress that we incur on a daily basis are aging us quicker than we should be aging. For one example, hormone levels are significantly lower at younger ages than in the past. I am seeing men and women with extremely low testosterone in their 30s and 40s, and I am seeing 40-year-old women who have the blood work of menopausal women. Why?

Aging is accentuated and accelerated by oxidative stress. Oxidative stress in the body is like pouring battery acid on something. It's caustic and causes decay, and the slow decay of our bodies is the definition of aging. Getting older means reduced function and the inability to ward off oxidative stressors, and, conversely, more oxidative stressors cause bodily functions to diminish and promote quicker aging. If you have picked up this book in good health, congratulations to you. By following the Freedom Diet suggestions and maintaining a good, balanced diet and lifestyle after the 60 days, you will age slower than your junk-eating, nonexercising, stressed-out counterpart.

PART 2

The Freedom Diet

The art of healing comes from nature,
not from the physician. Therefore, the
physician must start from nature,
with an open mind.

— PARACELSUS

CHAPTER 9

Changing Your Diet for Better Health

Paradigms of Medicine

Right now, at least two paradigms of healing exist in our society. One paradigm, which centers around diagnosing and treating disease, takes a mechanistic approach to illness in which the patient's symptoms are combated with pharmaceuticals and/or surgery. This approach assumes that if the patient's symptoms improve via painkillers, antibiotics, steroids, or other suppressive treatments, then the patient is cured.

Increasingly, our society is demanding a new paradigm of thought when approaching illness and the concept of wellness. People are looking for physicians who are less dogmatic and who provide tools and treatments that do more than just suppress symptoms. Thus, a second paradigm, the one embraced by naturopathic medicine, looks at the person as a whole and acts to stimulate his or her healing, even before disease is apparent. This paradigm, of which prevention is the cornerstone, strives to maintain homeostasis within the body, allowing it to function optimally and thereby promoting improved health.

Numerous studies support the fact that diet and lifestyle modifications improve health outcomes. For example, an article published in the *New England Journal of Medicine* in 2002 stated that diet and exercise may be more effective than pharmacologic therapy at defending against cardiovascular diseases in patients with impaired glucose tolerance. After three years of making diet and lifestyle changes, patients decreased their risk of developing diabetes by 58 percent. In contrast, participants who were only taking metformin, a common pharmaceutical prescription for diabetics, reduced their diabetes risk by only 31 percent—this is a significant difference. In addition, participants following the lifestyle changes had a significant reduction in C-reactive protein (CRP), which is an indirect marker of subclinical inflammation. Subclinical inflammation is inflammation that cannot be detected through the usual diagnostic procedures. Metformin participants affected their CRP levels significantly less than lifestyle-change participants.[71] These findings are huge breakthroughs for diabetic patients—if they get the information.

Another example of the effectiveness of dietary change on health was revealed in an article published in the *Canadian Medical Association Journal* in 2014, which supports the use of the Mediterranean diet for reversing metabolic syndrome.[72] The Freedom Diet and the Mediterranean diet have many similarities, but the Freedom Diet is more aggressive toward decreasing blood sugar and improving weight loss. Additionally, after the Freedom Diet I suggest that all patients continue on to the anti-inflammatory diet. The concept is simple: eat healthy vegetables, healthy fruits, healthy meats, and healthy fats, and keep your consumption of calorie-laden carbohydrates low.

Naturopathic physicians are recognized in some states as primary care physicians. In states where they are licensed to do so, naturopathic physicians provide lifestyle and diet-modification education in a primary care setting and actively teach prevention strategies. Naturopathic physicians offer dietary intervention, and many naturopathic physicians have seen their patients experience significant health improvements through diet and lifestyle change, as well as through various other naturopathic modalities. As a naturopathic physician, it is my duty and goal to educate my patients about how to change their overall health by changing their lifestyles.

I help put the power of healing into their hands. The body has an innate wisdom to heal itself, and sometimes it just needs a reminder to stimulate its own healing. We like to say that everyone has his or her own inner doctor, and a few wise choices in lifestyle habits can be a prescription for immensely improved quality of life. When we take better care of our vessels, they can be left to do amazing things on their own.

What Is Naturopathic Medicine?

A licensed naturopathic physician (ND) attends a four-year, graduate-level naturopathic medical school and is educated in all of the same basic sciences as a medical doctor (MD), with the difference being that he or she also studies holistic and nontoxic approaches to healing, with a strong emphasis on disease prevention and optimizing wellness. A naturopathic physician is board certified by his or her state and is expected to uphold the highest standards of primary medical care. Currently nineteen states are licensing naturopathic physicians. The licensed states are:

- Alaska
- Arizona
- California
- Colorado
- Connecticut
- District of Columbia
- Hawaii
- Kansas
- Maine
- Maryland
- Minnesota
- Montana
- New Hampshire
- North Dakota
- Oregon
- Utah
- Vermont

- Washington
- United States Territories: Puerto Rico and Virgin Islands

When searching for a naturopathic physician in states that do not have licensing procedures, it is important to find out about their credentials. In searching out a physician, make sure that you are being treated by a properly trained physician who has attended a four-year, accredited, postgraduate naturopathic medical school. There are currently eight accredited naturopathic medical schools in the United States and Canada. For more information about finding a naturopathic physician in your area, contact the American Association of Naturopathic Physicians or Canadian Association of Naturopathic Doctors.

Naturopathic medicine is successful at treating various acute and chronic diseases. The specialty excels in treating chronic illness, and many find relief when allopathic medicine has nothing left to offer. In acute conditions, naturopathic medicine often supports the body's own natural healing mechanism. Some common conditions treated by naturopathic medicine include, but are not limited to, allergies, asthma, anxiety, depression, fatigue, digestive complaints, skin complaints, autoimmune diseases, thyroid problems, menstrual irregularities (including menopause symptoms), acute colds and flus, chronic infections, and cancer.

As naturopathic physicians, we seek to help the body begin to restore health and maintain homeostasis. We pay attention to all aspects of the patient's body, mind, and spirit to ensure balance in all these areas. Often, simple dietary recommendations or a few lifestyle changes begin to turn the body around. At other times we need to help the body direct itself in a certain way by supporting specific systems with vitamins, minerals, botanicals, homeopathy, or other natural medicines.

Naturopathic physicians practice a system of therapy that relies on strict regimens of natural medicines to treat illness. According to the Coalition for Natural Health, naturopathic physicians historically "emphasized the use of hydrotherapy, nutrition, manipulation, herbs, or homeopathy[;] the goal for all practitioners of natural healing was to stimulate the body to heal itself. *Vis medicatrix naturae*, or the healing power of nature, remains central to naturopathic philosophy today." Rather than trying to attack specific diseases, natural doctors focus on cleansing and strengthening the body to bring about better wellness. Naturopathic medicine is founded on the following principles:

- The healing power of nature
- Do no harm
- Identify and treat the cause
- Treat the whole person
- Physician as teacher
- Prevention is the best cure
- Establish health and wellness

Methods and modalities are selected and applied based on these principles in relationship to the individual needs of the patient. Naturopathic medical practice utilizes all methods of clinical and laboratory diagnostic testing, including diagnostic radiology and other imaging techniques, blood work, pap smear testing, and various others. Naturopathic physicians can refer patients to specialists as needed. Like other health professionals, naturopathic physicians tend to specialize in one or a few conditions, but because naturopathic physicians treat the person rather than the illness, their scope is rather wide, and they can treat a large variety of illnesses.

Naturopathic medical treatment utilizes a variety of modalities, including but not limited to:

- dietary and lifestyle interventions
- botanical medicine
- homeopathy
- counseling
- naturopathic physician medicine, including injection therapies like prolotherapy and platelet-rich plasma
- vitamin and mineral therapy
- injection therapies, including neural therapy
- IV therapy

Naturopathic medicine involves distinct systems of primary care; it is an art, science, philosophy, and medical practice of diagnosis, treatment, and prevention of illness involving the whole body. The diagnosis by a naturopathic physician may go much deeper than the primary diagnosis. We may look into the causes of immune dysfunction, glandular weaknesses, organ insufficiencies, biochemistry imbalances, and so on to come up with a treatment plan that addresses all aspects of a patient's illness etiology.

In the development of personalized medicine, many contributing factors must be assessed, including one's environment, medical history, and upbringing, microbial balance, psychosomatic disorders, physical demands, additional health complaints, genetics, vitality, willingness to follow treatment and commitment to healing, hormone balance, etc. A skilled practitioner will be able to assess all of these factors and determine how and when to intervene with treatments and lifestyle changes.

Instead of merely suppressing symptoms, treatment of any condition must always be multifactorial to improve wellness. Natural treatment options available now are extensive, and the profusion of herbs, natural and over-the-counter medicines, and supplements that line the shelves of every store is overwhelming and confusing. Many times, having a plan created by a naturopathic physician, whose expertise is natural medicine, can help you gain wellness faster than trying to self-treat. Just taking everything off the shelf is not a good idea. Additionally, if you have an allopathic physician, they can help you with many issues, but you need someone other than the Internet to help guide you through a wellness plan involving extensive natural supplementation and lifestyle changes.

It is a bit presumptuous of me to claim that I can make a program that fits everyone, but after using this same diet plan and program for many individuals, I know that it will benefit everyone in some way if adopted completely. Many people lose weight, improve their blood sugar levels, feel better, have better energy, and feel like they have a new lease on life. All of these reasons are good ones for starting this important diet and lifestyle change.

Many people think that changing their diet is hard, and they simply don't want to make the effort to do it. Many think, *I have tried to diet before. I never lost any weight and I wasn't successful, so why try again.* I am here to tell you that this diet isn't necessarily about weight loss; it is about future health and making a significant enough change to improve your blood sugar balance and outcome for the future. It is also unfair to call permanent lifestyle changes a "diet." You want to make these changes and commit to a healthier collection of food choices for the rest of your life. If you can think of it like that, you are much more likely to be successful in your endeavors.

Additionally, adhering to this diet helps people age more gracefully, which I am always excited about. Consider that as you develop habits from this plan and maintain them for a long time, even beyond the 60 days, you will reduce how quickly you age as well as reducing future chronic disease risk. This of course refers to not only to the aging that we see on the outside, but also the aging that happens on the inside—to the blood vessels and all of the hidden, intricately networked organs. If you are diabetic and make this change, you may be saving yourself from many complications such as amputation or Alzheimer's disease.

Consider also that as you develop these lifelong habits, your freedom to do the things you couldn't before increases. You may be able to take longer walks, you may have more energy to spend time with your grandkids. Whatever positive effect you gain, it is well worth the sacrifice of avoiding the garbage and eating the good stuff, and well worth the time invested in exercising, food preparation, meditation, and improving your mental nutrition.

You Really Are What You Eat

The most important part of my practice in the development of a treatment plan with my patients is diet. You have probably heard the phrase "you are what you eat" a million times throughout your life. Have you ever stopped to think of what the phrase means or why it has become such a popular cliché?

Laws of physics state that every object or being can be broken down into smaller and smaller molecules. The smallest part that makes up any object or being is energy. Because all objects are made of energy, we can deduce that human beings are made wholly of energy. This also means that all food is energy. If we stopped eating energy-giving foods to fuel our body processes, we could not live for very long. That being said, doesn't it make sense to pay attention to what we consume each day? The food we eat is the fuel for all bodily processes. If you owned an extremely valuable car and wanted it to run at its optimal level, wouldn't you put the best-quality gas and oil into it? Likewise, if you value your body (and, accordingly, your health and your life), isn't it time to put the best-quality food or "fuel" into it?

Just as different objects have varying energy composition, different foods also have varying energies. We need to pay attention to the quality of food we put into our bodies. Food that is organically grown, freshly picked, and has spent the least amount of time in transport has the most vitality and therefore will offer you the highest-quality energy and nutrients. The more processing a food undergoes, the more toxins and the less energy and nutrient value it holds. Here's a general rule to remember: If you can't tell what a food is by looking at it, don't eat it. For example, white bread is made from wheat, but does it look like wheat? Can you tell it was made from wheat? Then you probably should not eat it.

Eating foods that are locally produced and in season is a great way to ensure good quality and good vitality. Foods that have been dehydrated, boxed for weeks or sometimes months, or canned in aluminum may be devoid of energy and full of preservatives, additives, and possibly dyes. These processed food items may offer a significantly reduced number of nutrients compared with fresh foods. Anything that is heat processed, dried, or powdered becomes significantly less healthy and significantly higher in compounds that cause oxidation in the body. A good example of dehydrated foods that are consumed often include dehydrated cheeses or milk products such as those found in crackers, mixes, hot cocoa, boxed macaroni and cheese, and many other instant items.

We can obtain some vital micronutrients (vitamins, minerals, and phytochemicals), which are used to support metabolism and energy, through supplementation, but the macronutrients needed to fuel the body (carbohydrates, proteins, and fats) can only come from food. Because the food we eat is our only source of fuel, we really are what we eat. Eating food out of cans day after day may leave a person feeling fatigued and devoid of energy, similar to the energy of the food he or she is consuming.

Our diet should be composed of real food, but that is not what most people in our society are consistently eating. The Freedom Diet is not easy, but it is extremely rewarding and has helped many of my patients to get control over their lives and to feel well again. Some of my patients have done incredible things with their lives after following this diet. Many type 2 diabetics have reversed the disease and gotten their blood sugars back to normal by adopting these diet and lifestyle practices. Examples of whole foods that should be included in the diet are fresh vegetables, fresh berries (we avoid most fruits at first, but don't worry, you can add them back in later), very limited grains (always soaked prior to cooking), limited legumes (also soaked prior to cooking), and clean meats such as lamb, buffalo, grass-fed ground beef, and free-range, organic chicken or turkey.

Also include plenty of filtered water. You should be drinking half your weight in ounces in filtered water daily. That means if you weigh 300 pounds then, yes, you should be drinking 150 ounces per day. Filtered water is important. The foods that are important to consume on this diet facilitate a direct purpose: reversing how your body processes sugar in the diet. Your GI tract breaks down all food into blood glucose to transport to cells for energy. If you are diabetic, are prediabetic, or merely want to lose weight or slow the aging process, this diet will refocus the metabolism to store sugars properly and improve the glucose–insulin response.

It is impossible in a book to fine-tune a diet to fit everyone; therefore, take some of these suggestions with a grain of salt. For example, if you are unable to eat avocados because you had a reaction in the past, merely omit them from your diet. I have also described how to eliminate foods and reintroduce them at a later date so that you become more familiar with the foods that may be plaguing you.

Elimination and Challenge Method

Several methods exist to test for food intolerances or allergies. The true gold standard is an elimination and challenge diet. If a person is very diligent, this approach can be an inexpensive and very effective approach to discovering food allergies or intolerances.

The best way to implement the elimination and challenge diet is to strictly eliminate a food or combination of foods for at least four to eight weeks. After that time, each food that you have eliminated can be introduced individually in its most whole form. For example, if you were avoiding tomatoes because you wanted to reduce inflammation, then you can introduce them at a later date. To introduce tomatoes, eat one whole tomato after avoiding anything with tomatoes for at least four weeks; do not eat tomato sauce, ketchup, or tomato soup. After eating the tomato, don't eat any more tomatoes or tomato products for three days because some reactions may be delayed. After three days, assuming you've had no reaction to the tomato, you can probably assume that tomatoes are a safe food for you and you can start eating them again, but still not daily. Then after one week you can introduce the next food in its whole form, wait three days, and so on. If you have a reaction immediately, then you can assume that the food you introduced is not good for you and you should avoid it. Since you've already shown a reaction to the recently introduced food, you may introduce the next food without waiting the usual one week. A common example of a reaction to reintroducing tomatoes occurs when an arthritic person had improvement in arthritis symptoms when not consuming tomatoes, but then has a recurrence of stiffness and pain after reintroducing tomatoes into the diet.

If you have a hard time strictly eliminating a number of foods, instead eliminate and then reintroduce one food at a time. For example, avoid all dairy products for one month, including butter and cream (although they are listed on my approved foods). Then reintroduce them by drinking one glass of milk, and wait up to three days for any reaction. Then eliminate the next food, and so on.

Usually, reactions come in the form of something you have experienced before. This is your area of weakness or susceptibility. For example, reintroducing dairy may cause sinus issues in one person, reflux in a baby, constipation in another person, and a migraine in someone else. For another example, if one is prone to migraines, then a migraine may occur; if one is prone to diarrhea or digestive distress, then diarrhea may occur. Reactions are not limited to susceptible systems, however, and can be anything from mild congestion to mood disturbance to severe abdominal cramps. Some reactions may be immediate and some may be delayed; that is why we have individuals wait up to one week before introducing the next food.

After following the elimination and challenge diet, one may learn what types of foods he or she reacts to. It has been my experience and observation, however, that for someone with a chronic disease, following the diet the way it is presented will offer the best optimal health. For example, it is recommended that chronically ill patients avoid all gluten—even organic whole wheat and even if no reaction is noted during the elimination and challenge phase of the diet—until their health improves and their terrain is treated.

Foods to Include

Vegetables	Fruits	Proteins	Nuts/ Seeds/ Legumes	Fats	Drinks/ Seasonings
kale	raspberries	wild salmon	garbanzo beans	avocado	organic coffee
collard greens	blueberries	organic chicken	lentils, split peas, dal	homemade mayo (egg, oil, mustard)	organic tea
chard	blackberries	organic turkey	white beans	cream – small amount used in coffee/tea	water, filtered or bottled
broccoli	strawberries	organic lamb	chia seeds	organic butter	vinegar
cabbage	cherries	organic grass-fed beef	flax seeds	coconut	herbs and spices
celery	rhubarb	hor-mone-free eggs	salba seeds	full-fat coconut milk (mild heat only)	soy sauce, gluten free and unsweet-ened
carrot	lemon		sunflower seeds, raw and unsalted	olive oil (mild heat only)	unsweetened lemon juice

beets, raw	lime		pumpkin seeds, raw and unsalted	coconut oil	unsweetened lime juice
peas, fresh			hemp hearts	flaxseed oil (do not heat)	unsweetened almond milk
sweet potato			quinoa	hempseed oil (do not heat)	unsweetened hemp milk
yams					unsweetened flax milk
tomatoes					yacon syrup or flakes
radish					stevia
parsley					garlic
cauliflower					ginger
red pepper					turmeric
yellow pepper					
green pepper					
cucumber					
onion					
green onion					
brussels sprout					
spinach					
asparagus					
green beans					
romaine lettuce					
red- and green-leaf lettuce					
butter lettuce					
mushrooms					

mustard greens					
summer squash					
leeks					
sauerkraut, raw					
artichoke					

Foods to Avoid

Based on reading this text so far, you may guess what I am going to say to avoid. This might be very different for many of you, especially insulin users who are used to being able to carb count and then combat your carb intake with your insulin dose. I am asking you to be extremely consistent and compliant with this plan for the next 60 days so you can begin to understand the freedom that you can gain with this diet. If you are on insulin, please ask your physician for help so that you are able to monitor your insulin dosage along with your blood sugars. Oftentimes, people need much less insulin rather quickly while starting this diet. If you are not on insulin but are on a diabetic medication, also consider visiting your physician to inquire about a plan for the use of your medication alongside this optimal health plan.

There is a long list of offending foods that should be avoided. What I want you to concentrate more on is what you can eat. Think about the meals you can enjoy, and begin to experiment in your own kitchen. Get a friend to do this with you. You don't have to be prediabetic or diabetic to follow this diet; you merely have to want to improve your health, maybe lose some weight, feel better, have more energy, and have less risk for chronic health issues in the future. If you have any inflammation at all, it is extremely gratifying to test your inflammatory markers before and after this plan so that you can feel the overwhelming sense of accomplishment when you see your numbers begin to improve.

Foods to Avoid

Vegetables	Fruits	Proteins	Nuts/ Seeds/ Legumes	Fats	Drinks/ Seasonings
parsnips	mango	nonorganic meats	all grains, such as corn, wheat, rice, oats	fried foods	juice
potatoes, red, white, yellow, purple	watermelon	hormone-containing meats	all other legumes	canola oil	vegetable juices
canned vegetables	oranges		all nuts and nut butters	grapeseed oil	soda
rutabaga	grapefruit		popcorn	sunflower oil	sweetened drinks like tea
beets, cooked	papaya		polenta	safflower oil	coffee drinks
Jerusalem artichoke	apples		cereals		alcohol
	cantaloupe				energy drinks
	grapes, green and red				all sugar
	cranberry				chocolate
	pineapple				maple syrup
	peaches				agave syrup
	persimmon				honey
	kiwi				all added sweeteners*
	bananas				
	canned fruits				

*I have listed names of added sweeteners here: maltodextrin, maltose, dextrose, glucose, sucrose, trehalose, inverted sugar, high-fructose corn syrup, HFCS-42, HFCS-55, and HFCS-90 (forms of high-fructose corn syrup), caramel, golden syrup, refiners syrup, blackstrap molasses, maple syrup, honey, sorghum syrup, lactose, cane juice, barley malt syrup, hydrogenated starch hydrolysate (HSH), coconut palm sugar, maltitol, brown rice syrup, fructose, galactose, agave syrup, xylitol, glycerol, sorbitol, lactitol, isomalt, mannitol, erythritol, acesulfame potassium (Ace K), alitame, aspartame (NutraSweet, Equal), sodium cyclamate, neotame, saccharin (Sweet'n Low), and sucralose (Splenda).

CHAPTER 10

Habits to Include

Our habits can truly help improve our health outcomes. Our habits brought us to our current state of health, but we have the power to change them. It is never too late to make significant health changes, and it is never too late to start with improved diet and lifestyle habits. The habits that I am going to list below I have suggested to thousands and thousands of patients over the years, and I have seen significant benefits in those who make the choice to follow all of the recommendations. Be strict with yourself, create a challenge for yourself, and see yourself accomplish it.

The Freedom Diet and lifestyle plan is set up as a 60-day plan, but I am hoping that you follow it long enough to help you create a habit that is lifelong. Remember that numerous studies support what I am about to present to you in terms of the important lifestyle changes you should make for improved future health. What motivates me to stay in shape and eat well is my children. I want to be active and healthy for them as they get older, as well as for my future grandchildren. I want to be a role model for them and want to be a role model for my patients. I can't ask them to undertake a significant diet change without myself also being able to do it. I can't ask them to incorporate exercise and sleep if I won't do it myself. This is not to portray myself as a holy do-gooder all of the time. I make mistakes, I cheat every once in a while, I might miss a day of exercise, but healthy eating, sleeping, and exercise have become my norm and that is important. When they become your habit, if you cheat or fall off, it is extremely easy to get back on and stay on for life. I consider it staying on the path toward better health or enlightenment with small bumps, or pit stops, along the way.

Here are some very important habits to create:

- sleep
- exercise
- meditation or stress relief
- nutrition for the mind
- water intake
- dietary hygiene

Sleep

The goal is for you to sleep more than seven hours per night. If you are not sleeping upwards of seven to eight hours nightly, chronic disease risks increase. If it is simply because you don't go to bed early enough and have to get up early in the morning, try going to bed to allow yourself time to get eight hours of sleep for two to three months straight. You will be surprised at what changes you see. If your goal is weight loss, remember that getting eight hours of sleep nightly is key to your weight loss program.

Remove media from the bedroom, and sleep in complete darkness every night. Make sure you are not using media for one hour prior to going to bed, as this will help you calm down before heading to bed. Sleeping in complete darkness is extremely important, as it will help the body naturally produce more melatonin, the hormone that promotes sleep. Melatonin does an incredible amount more than help us sleep, as we discussed previously.

I suggest blackout curtains to help improve the darkness of the room. If you find after your room is completely dark that you have a difficult time waking up in the morning, consider getting a wake light. These are easy to find on Amazon.com or elsewhere on the Internet and gradually lighten until the time you set the alarm, so they naturally promote your body's reduced production of melatonin, helping you rise easier.

Go to bed earlier. For every hour you sleep before midnight, something powerful seems to happen. For my patients who regularly don't get to sleep until after midnight, regardless of how late they sleep in the morning, healing is slower from a clinical perspective. I tell most of my adult patients that they should go to bed at 10:00 p.m. For most people's schedules, that allows plenty of time to get seven or eight hours of sleep.

If you have a sleep disorder, it is very important that you spend some time at the doctor's office figuring it out. If you have been diagnosed with sleep apnea, using a CPAP mask can improve daily energy and nightly sleep. If you have not had your mask adjusted or have stopped using it due to inconvenience, I encourage you to visit your doctor again as the CPAP masks have been improved for patient comfort.

If you are unable to fall asleep and do not have sleep apnea, you may find improved sleep after adopting the diet and starting exercise and meditation. If you are still not sleeping well, consider a visit to your doctor to optimize your sleep habits while you are doing this 60-day program, as you are better able to lose weight and improve blood sugar levels while you are sleeping well.

You also can try taking a spoonful of almond butter at night before bed to balance blood sugar levels throughout the night. This boost of fat and protein works to prevent rebound cortisol increases from blood sugar imbalance.

My complete list of recommendations for sleep is as follows:

- Sleep over seven hours nightly.
- Sleep in a completely dark room.
- Go to bed earlier.
- Get evaluated for sleep disorders and treat them if needed.
- Make sure your surroundings are conducive to restful sleep. If you use your cell phone as an alarm clock, make sure incoming calls and text messages are silenced, and distance the phone from your head.
- Keep your room cool, and invest in a good mattress.
- Consider using sleep-enhancing supplements such as magnesium, GABA, L-theanine, 5-HTP, or melatonin
- Manage your stress well during the day, include regular daily

exercise, and maintain a regular routine throughout the day.
- Consider a nightly meditation or prayer to calm your nerves for a restful night.

Exercise

Picture exercise as a prescription from your doctor. Instead of having to take the small capsule, however, you take up exercise and you do it well. Everyone should work themselves up to a robust but safe exercise program. I suggest getting a trainer to help you if you have significant health complaints. For the average healthy individual, I suggest starting at 30 minutes three times per week and working your way up to 45–60 minutes at least four to five days per week. Essentially, if we did it the way nature intended, we should exercise every day we eat! So according to that plan, our exercise should be daily, but don't beat yourself up if you can't make it every day. Make an effort to get there "nearly" every day.

If you are new to and unfamiliar with exercise and don't know your level of fitness, you can start with 10 minutes every day. It can be brisk walking, climbing up and down the stairs, doing yoga, riding a bike or stationary bike, or swimming. With the ever-increasing number of exercise activities out there, you have plenty of exercise activities to choose from. Make sure you have a visit with your physician to discuss your new exercise program before beginning.

Because I don't know you and cannot see you during a physician visit, I do not understand your physique or what types of exercise you will do best with. I do know that exercise is vital to this program as it is vital to improved health and prevention of chronic illness. The body wants to know it is alive, and exercise is a great way to tell your physical body that you are still in it to win it.

Consider a balance between weight-bearing exercises and muscle-strengthening exercises. Weight-bearing exercises can be considered exercises that use the body and exert the body's force upon its own muscles and joints. Muscle-strengthening exercises involve using weights during the workout with the goal of strengthening the muscle. High-impact weight-bearing exercises help build bones and keep them strong. These exercises may not be right for everyone, especially those with degenerative joint disease or previous fractures. Low-impact weight-bearing exercises can be a great alternative for someone who is not able to do the high-impact exercises. Low-impact exercises will still help keep bones and joints healthy. Obviously, all of the exercises listed below may not be right for everyone, and if you have never done these exercises before, I suggest meeting with a trainer for guidance before initiating.

Examples of high-impact weight-bearing exercises are:

- dancing
- hiking
- doing high-impact aerobics
- jogging/running
- jumping rope
- jumping jacks
- stair climbing or using the stair climber at the gym on high setting
- tennis

Examples of low-impact weight-bearing exercises are:

- elliptical training machines
- low-impact aerobics
- yoga with strength poses
- hula hooping
- stair climber machine on slow setting
- mat pilates
- slow to fast walking on a treadmill or outside

Examples of muscle-strengthening exercises are:

- lifting weights
- using elastic exercise bands
- doing lunges or squats while holding weights
- using weight machines
- lifting your own body weight
- pilates on the reformer machine (need supervision/class)

- functional movements, such as standing and rising up on your toes

If you are already exercising, in good shape, and uninjured, then begin by increasing the length of time you exercise by 20 percent. Studies reveal that no matter how much you are exercising now, increasing by 20 percent can help reduce blood sugar and manage diabetes easier. Adding weight-bearing and muscle-strengthening exercises daily can also help the body maintain better-balanced blood sugar levels. If you are currently already lifting, gradually increase the amount of weight you are lifting by 20 percent.

If you are not exercising but are in good shape and uninjured, then begin exercising every day consistently at the same time of day. I believe exercising every day is the best exercise habit we can adopt. I suggest beginning with seven- to ten-minute workouts daily and then increasing from there.

If you want to go to the gym, you can start with 10 minutes of cardio exercise on the elliptical, treadmill, stair climber, bike, or other machine you like. If you like swimming, you can start swimming for 10 minutes every day. If you cannot go to a gym and don't want to exercise to videos, then get out and speed walk or jog.

After initiating exercise, the goal will be to increase the amount of time you spend exercising gradually until you reach at least 30–60 minutes daily and maintain that every day for the rest of your life. Obviously, there are going to be times that we miss, or maybe our daily activities only allow us to regularly exercise four to five times per week. According to research, exercising daily can reduce our risk for premature death by a significant percentage.

If you are not exercising, not in good shape, or injured, then consult a physical trainer. I cannot express strongly enough how much working with a trainer can help you. I have had physical trainers from time to time and still use some of the exercises that I learned from them. They can help you devise a plan that will keep you safe as you increase your level of activity. They can help you prevent future injury and even strengthen the areas that are weak to potentially improve any injuries that you have. Start slow and try to exercise daily. If you meet with your trainer once per week, ask them to help you make a plan so that when your trainer is not there, you are able to safely do the exercises on your own.

Try to manage at least 10 minutes per day. Obviously, on the days you are with your trainer, you may exercise longer because you will be discussing and assessing your needs to develop a personalized plan.

After initiating exercise, the goal will be to increase the amount of time you spend exercising gradually until you reach at least 30–60 minutes daily and maintain that every day for the rest of your life. Obviously, there are going to be times that we miss, or maybe our daily activities only allow us to regularly exercise four to five times per week. According to research, exercising daily can reduce our risk for premature death by a significant percentage.

Meditation or Stress Relief

Here is a simple meditation technique. It is called mindfulness. Sitting upright in a chair with your feet on the ground or beneath you is a great place to start. You want to be comfortable but not lounging. Set a timer on your phone or other device, and lay it beside you. Begin by closing your eyes, keeping good posture, and taking a deep breath in. The idea behind mindfulness meditation is to clear the mind. When you are new to meditating, your mind will be extremely active when you meditate. I still get some of my best ideas while I am trying to meditate. As you breathe in and out, try your best to concentrate on your breath. Take a breath in and a breath out, and try to keep them deep and slow. There is no need to count and no need to stress.

Mindfulness means nonjudgment. Don't judge what you think you are going to get from the meditation, don't judge yourself and how you meditate, don't judge yourself when your mind is all over the place. After you have taken some deep breaths, try to clear your mind. What you will find is that a lot of thoughts will come up, and it is best to just categorize them and move on. It might be an "idea" thought or a "to do" thought or a "judgment" thought about yourself or others. Just realize that your mind is no longer on your breath, take note of the thought, and release it. Go back to thinking about your breathing.

When I first started this practice, my mind wandered the entire time, and oftentimes still does. Maybe I haven't mastered the technique yet, but what I do know is that sometimes I do a lot of processing during these quiet times. I can think clearer, develop unique ideas, and make better decisions if I commit to spending time in a meditative state. When you begin, start with only five minutes per day, because anyone can afford five minutes in a day if they set their mind to it. Do not open your eyes until your timer goes off. My challenge to you is to increase by five more minutes each week or at least every two weeks. By the end of the 60-day program, you could be spending 20–40 minutes per day meditating. It is not a terribly long commitment of time, especially when we know the health benefits that result from meditating, which we discussed in chapter 1.

Mindfulness meditation is only one form of meditation out of many. Transcendental meditation has been extensively studied, and the people I have met who practice it have the most amazing, calming presence about them. I haven't learned it but from what I know, it can be extremely beneficial for anyone who wants to try, and it is extremely easy to learn. You will have to contact a transcendental meditation teacher in your area, as the way you learn is through a hands-on teacher-to-student program. I am longing to do this in the future.

Nutrition for the Mind

Begin thinking positive thoughts daily. Check in with yourself a couple of times per day and see how happy you are. This helps to keep you accountable. Also, you can do various things to keep your mind focused on positive thoughts. One idea is to have positive sayings posted around your house such as on your mirror, in your car, at your desk, etc. Make sure the people you surround yourself with are positive and make you feel good about yourself. Limit the time you spend around negative people, and when conversations are negative, make an effort to switch them to something positive. All you have to do is take the same thing the person is talking about and say something positive about it. You will be surprised at how much you can change a conversation if you pay attention and are aware of it.

I also think you need to consider what type of brain nutrition you are offering yourself. Consider that everything you allow yourself to be stimulated by mentally or emotionally stimulates neurotransmitters in your brain. Therefore, watching the news, laden with negativity, every night before bed can affect what your subconscious mind is processing during sleep. Additionally, frequently watching violent television shows or movies validates that type of feeling or behavior, and you will have more of a tendency to exhibit that behavior or aggression. This is especially true for children. When children are bombarded with negative media, video games, and violent movies, their attitudes can reflect the type of mental and emotional stimuli they are taking in on a daily basis.

Similarly, watching funny movies, talking about lighthearted subjects, daydreaming about a positive, happy future, and spending time with others doing positive things can promote a more positive feeling about yourself. I know that when I have a great day of seeing patients, I feel better. On the days that all of my patients are feeling better and we can laugh and feel good together, at the end of the day I feel incredible. On the flip side, I have harder days when many of my patients are not doing well or not feeling well and there is no laughing. At the end of such a day, I feel exhausted and less positive.

Volunteering your time with others can be such a rewarding way to feel surrounded by more positive people. My daughter and I spend a lot of time volunteering together for various philanthropies, and what I have found is that I feel incredible after whatever volunteer project we have just finished, whether it is helping those in need get food or clothes, reading books to kids, planting trees, or spending time helping with the Special Olympics. What I have found is that the other people you volunteer with have the brightest hearts and the most inviting smiles, and I love being around people who are willing to spend their time helping others.

The moral of the story is to find something that you can do often that makes you feel good and that is a positive habit for you and those around you. When you begin to feel happier, your health improves. When you are happier, so are the people around you, so make an effort to bring up your level of happiness.

Positive Affirmations

One form of positive affirmation is to say something out loud to yourself to make yourself feel better. It is a way you can slowly retrain the subconscious to think a little differently. Positive affirmations can have a large impact on your self-esteem and self-worth. Improving your self-worth is vital to healing, because if you have good self-worth, you will want to take care of your body and take care of your health. You value yourself and want to keep yourself in shape if you love yourself. Here are a few quick sentences you can say to yourself on a daily basis:

- I completely love and accept myself.
- I am healthy, energetic, and happy.
- I am connected to my community and feel good.
- I feel positive and loving toward myself and others.

Obviously these are just ideas, and you can use other ideas to formulate your own positive affirmations. They may be directed at your health or your being, but should not be directed at any monetary or possession gains. Additionally, when formulating your own affirmation sentence, you should frame it in the positive form rather than the negative one. Don't use words like *don't*, *won't*, and *not*, and don't use words that represent ill health. I have listed a couple of examples below and have followed them with improved positive affirmations. Finally, all positive affirmations should be said in present tense. Saying them in any other tense, even future tense, is like admitting that you don't feel that way.

Examples of inadequate affirmations:

- I don't have diabetes anymore.
- I won't think negative thoughts about myself and others anymore.
- I am cancer free.
- I won't think negative thoughts.

Improved affirmations:

- My blood sugars are balanced and healthy.
- I completely love myself and others.
- I am healthy and vibrant.
- I think clearly and positively.

Other Forms of Stress Relief

Stress and a lack of mental/emotional wellness are huge contributors to illness and inflammation. Chronic stress, cynical distrust, and depression were linked with elevated levels of inflammatory markers in a large cross-sectional study published a few years ago in the journal *Archives of Internal Medicine*.[73] Numerous other studies support the finding that negative emotions increase inflammatory markers and contribute to poor health. When we are under stress, our bodies secrete the same chemicals that trigger inflammation.

Calming the brain is important. Calming the body is important. Reducing stress is important. Almost everyone knows by now that stress can cause disease and can eventually kill, but many do nothing about it, continuing to live their day-to-day lives in turmoil. This doesn't have to be the case. There are simple solutions for stress reduction that needn't take up too much time in your busy schedule. Learning to balance your stress with lighthearted happiness is important enough to prioritize.

Here are some simple pointers for reducing stress and finding calm:

- Breathe. Concentrate on taking deep breaths into the belly. Do this throughout the day, or spend five minutes in the morning or evening sitting up straight, with good posture, breathing. This is similar to the meditating practice described above but can sometimes feel less intimidating or overwhelming if I describe it as just breathing.
- Exercise or get outside daily.
- Obtain counseling, if needed.
- Develop a community of people you can talk to and spend time with. Developing a community of people

who support your important lifestyle changes and who also want to have or adopt healthy habits is especially important. Just learning new health or cooking tips from others can reduce your stress when you are faced with planning your meals or exercise habits.

- Spend one to three minutes every day thinking positive thoughts and visualizing what you want. Some spiritual traditions teach that our bodies don't distinguish between good feelings generated by our imaginations and those that come from actually experiencing something pleasant. I often suggest to my patients that they visualize themselves sitting in beautiful surroundings experiencing vibrant health. This goes along with keeping a positive mind. Just keeping yourself feeling more positive will help you limit stress levels.

- Laugh out loud. Watch funny movies. Limit your TV watching to shows that make you feel good, not stressed or depressed.

- Pet your dog or cat. A companion animal's unconditional love can immediately make you feel calmer.

- Clean out the clutter from your surroundings. Make sure your bedroom is uncluttered and is simply and pleasingly decorated.

- Listen to music or sing a song. The right type of music can be very healing for some people. Listening to music that triggers memories of a very happy time in your life can often improve mood and decrease stress.

- Write in your journal. It's like venting without having to have someone around who can listen to you. Journaling forces you to process your thoughts as you are writing them down. You can even do a ritual of burning each page after you write it so that you feel the tension ease as the stressful event you just wrote about is lifted into the air.

- Take supplements that support your adrenal glands. B vitamins and magnesium are two of the best supplements for aiding adrenal function; taking them regularly can help a person feel significantly less fatigued.

- If you're in a healthy, committed relationship, have sex! I understand that sex may be the last thing on your mind, but you'll find that it helps improve feelings of well-being every time, and it helps to increase your natural testosterone and oxytocin, hormones that will help you feel more vital and connected to your community. Sex lowers blood pressure, boosts self-esteem, and increases feelings of intimacy with your partner.[74]
- Try taking alternating hot and cold showers. One of our patients shared with us a trick he learned after a few years of marriage. He takes a hot and then a cold shower right before bedtime. It revives his energy, makes his body feel tingly, and makes him want to touch his wife. He reports that this regimen has dramatically improved his sex life—as well as his marriage in general. Additionally, alternating hot and cold showers helps to increase circulation, increase lymphatic detoxification, decrease inflammation, and improve elimination through the skin. It can help to relieve sinus congestion, break up mucus in upper respiratory infections, and stimulate glandular function. You can do a similar treatment using a hot tub or sauna in place of a hot shower. Make sure to always end with a cold rinse; this will carry blood back to your vital organs and close your pores so that you don't get a chill.

Water Intake

Drink half of your weight in ounces of filtered, clean water daily. Drinking water is extremely important to the daily functioning of your cells. The amount is easy to calculate. The average 150-pound person should drink 75 fluid ounces per day of water. I find that on the days that I am very consistent with water drinking, my energy is better and I crave foods less. If you weigh a lot, it can be surprising how much water your body needs. I still stand by this with my 300-pound patients; they should drink 150 ounces of water daily. At first this habit is hard, but if one can maintain this habit daily, weight loss is much easier.

Water and weight loss are directly connected, so if one of your goals is to lose weight, you must drink the amount of water I suggest. I have put many people on weight loss plans, and almost always if someone isn't drinking enough water, their body isn't able to lose the weight. The solution to pollution is dilution. Oftentimes, we need a healthy water-drinking habit to make sure we continually flush our bodies of toxins. When you are not drinking enough water, your body still wants to dilute the toxicity burden that it has to deal with. A smart solution the body has come up with in some people is adding extra adipose tissue. Remember what I mentioned earlier: everything the body does is to survive longer in its environment. So if the solution to pollution is dilution and you are not using water as your diluter, then your body has to come up with another solution, and that is often fat tissue.

All of the functions in your body are dependent on cell-to-cell communication. Cells have to be extremely close to each other to communicate, otherwise their messages don't get through. Oftentimes, cells touching each other can facilitate the right form of cell-to-cell stimulation. At any rate, our cells are surviving within a liquid and fluid environment. To maintain fluidity of cellular reaction, we want the cells to be able to freely move around and maintain cell-to-cell connections. I use a little analogy to talk to my patients about how important drinking water is for the body. I let my patients know that if they are drinking an adequate amount of water, we can picture their cells as grapes floating around communicating with each other. If people are not drinking enough water, then it is like raisins trying to float around and communicate with each other. I can imagine that raisins would just sink and not be very fluid. So then I ask my patients if they would rather have their cells be like grapes floating around communicating with each other or raisins trying to communicate.

Dietary Hygiene

Chew Your Food

Make sure to chew your food many, many times before swallowing. One main problem with the way we eat today is that we are eating way too fast. When we eat too fast, we don't allow our natural satiety signaling to catch up with how much food we have ingested. Additionally, not chewing our food well because we are eating too quickly can cause digestive problems and increase esophageal reflux. I suggest everyone try to sit down while eating during this 60-day plan and make sure you have time to chew your food. When people chew their food slowly at every bite, they tend to eat less. Try to chew your food around 21 times before swallowing. Obviously this is an arbitrary number and should be adjusted with the different foods you are eating. The goal of chewing well is to break the food particles into a very mushy consistency before swallowing. If you are having to force yourself to swallow food while you are eating by first bringing your chin down and then bringing your chin up through an arc while finally lifting your chin to swallow, you are swallowing your food before you have had a chance to adequately chew it. It is surprising how many overweight people are not chewing their foods properly. Check in with yourself while eating to make sure you are chewing well with every meal.

Don't Drink Anything While Eating

Drinking a lot of fluids while you eat can inhibit how effectively you are able to digest the food once it is in your stomach. Some people suggest drinking a lot of water before eating to help with weight loss or help you eat less with the meal, but I disagree with this suggestion for digestion purposes. If you want to make sure you eat less at a meal, I would suggest keeping extremely well-hydrated through the day and then drinking 12–24 ounces of water about an hour before the meal. This will help keep you from overeating.

You can take small sips of water during a meal to, as I would say, "wet the whistle," but no large gulps, and don't drink your entire serving of water after the meal. Give your body some time to digest the meal before you put a lot of water into your system. I suggest waiting at least 30 minutes after a meal and an hour if you ate a larger meal.

Ritual

Have a ritual you follow around your meals. This doesn't need to take a long time, but it does help you connect with the food as a part of your health plan rather than treating it as just a means to an end. It could be a silent prayer of thanks or it could be even taking three nice, long, deep breaths before you eat. You can say a prayer out loud with the people you are eating with. You can also consider putting your fork down in between each bite to take in one nice long breath, followed by a long breath out.

Family Meals

Family meals are extremely important for children and teenagers. Eating together with the family has been shown to decrease behavioral problems in teens. According to the National Center on Addiction and Substance Abuse at Columbia University, children who don't regularly eat dinner with their families are almost four times more likely to use tobacco, and over twice as likely to use alcohol or illegal drugs.[75] Setting boundaries with your children and teaching them good habits by example is the first step in raising well-adjusted young people.

Let's face it, everyone has problems, and families struggle with time demands and commitments, but maintaining routine and rhythm whenever possible can help ensure that your children understand who they are and what type of family they come from. It is important to teach them what your family values. I commonly repeat sayings to my children such as, "As a family, we eat well. As a family, we eat together on Wednesdays and Sundays. As a family, we are courteous to others. As a family, we don't eat candy. As a family, we eat our vegetables." You get the point. Teaching children who they are is important, but we can't just say it, we have to live it if we want our children to follow our example.

I was taking my child into school today and she said to me, "Megan's mom is healthy too." I didn't understand initially what this meant, as I hadn't met Megan or her mom. I asked my daughter how she knew this and she said, "Because she brings a healthy lunch also." I asked her if it looked good and she said yes. Then I asked her if she would like to eat what was in Megan's lunch and she said, "No, I want what is in my lunch, but I think you should meet Megan's mom because you would like her." She hadn't even met her, but she understood that health was an important aspect of her family and that joining with others in the community with similar values is beneficial. I was very proud of this comment because sometimes it is hard to be different, and I understand that her lunch, to most of her classmates, is probably not appetizing, but it is what my daughter has grown up with and has become her norm, and I can guarantee that she will be packing healthy lunches for her children when she grows up.

I bring this point up because it is hard to be different, no matter what your age is. So if everyone at work is snacking on the candy and chips in the lunchroom, it is difficult to be the person who always brings salad. But I can guarantee you that if you set the example, some may follow, and if you do it continually for years in the same workplace, you will start to see the differences between your health and the health of those around you who continually consume the wrong foods and follow the wrong lifestyle patterns.

Eat Breakfast

Eating breakfast every day is extremely important. If you are one of those people who are extremely hungry at dinnertime and end up eating many of your calories then, you are most likely not eating enough during the day. Making sure that you eat a balanced breakfast in the morning leads to weight loss, more satiety, and balanced blood sugar levels throughout the day. If you are feeling really hungry by noon, then you may not be eating enough for breakfast, so use this as your gauge and increase your protein, fat, and veggies at breakfast.

Snacking can be a great way to prevent blood sugar spikes and drops throughout the day. I suggest a small protein and/or vegetable snack between meals. Your goal is to eat about every two hours. I am not a calorie counter, but you want to keep these snacks small. They are not meant to take the place of a meal, and if you eat too large of a snack, then you may not have the proper appetite balance for your other meals. Aim for about 150 calories. There are many food apps to help you count calories, and you are welcome to sign up for my portal as well so you can track your blood sugar, blood pressure, weight, what you are eating, and much more. See details in the list of recommended websites at the end of the book.

Here is a list of some tasty snacks that are approved on the Freedom Diet:

- snap peas
- raw sliced peppers
- raw yellow beet with hummus
- any vegetable you are able to eat raw
- celery with sunflower butter
- romaine lettuce with hummus
- romaine lettuce wrapped around steamed chicken
- romaine lettuce wrapped around chunk light tuna or canned salmon
- spinach leaves with hummus
- hard-boiled egg
- avocado with spinach or romaine leaves
- green drink (see recipes)
- organic, plain, whole-fat yogurt with berries (omit if dairy intolerant)
- organic, plain, whole-fat cottage cheese with berries (omit if dairy intolerant)
- chicken salad on butter lettuce

CHAPTER 11

Habits to Avoid

Here are some very important habits to avoid:

- watching television
- negative thinking
- spending time with unhealthy people
- toxic exposure
- self-medicating with substances
- overeating

Watching Television

There are numerous studies linking sedentary behavior to increased risk for chronic illness, inflammation, type 2 diabetes, and premature death. Keep your TV watching or Internet surfing to less than one hour per day. You can think of this as cumulative weekly, as you may not watch anything for three nights in a row but then sit down with a friend or loved one to watch a movie together. This is fine as long as the television doesn't become your every-night activity. Active people stay healthier longer. If your job requires you to be at a computer all day, make sure you exercise and take breaks in the day to look up, get up, and stretch your body. And I would suggest that if you are sitting down at the computer all day, you limit your television use to almost none. Find different activities for the evenings, go places, sign up for a class or a sport, go for a walk, do anything but sit sedentarily.

Negative Thinking

This goes back to thinking more about what mental and emotional nutrition we bring into our bodies. You certainly must create the habit of positivity. This will help you immensely when developing your future health habits. If you find yourself complaining, stop and stay something nice about what you are complaining about and then just let it go; it will feel a lot better than continuing to brood. Avoid people who are complaining or doing negative things as well.

Brooding is a common and undermining form of negativity. A person will take any situation that has happened in the near or distance past and continue to dwell on it. This can happen for various reasons. It may be because they would have liked to act differently or for a situation to turn out different than it did. They may think they were wronged by another person or treated unfairly. Whatever it is, if you are brooding about something, whether a previous relationship or a problem, it is time to let things go. You can do this by various methods, including counseling, meditation, hypnotherapy, and other means. Journaling can be a great way to let something go. After you are done with the journal, burn the pages and allow yourself to be free of the issue. You can do this any time you start to brood about the problem again. You need to accept that you cannot change what has happened in the past but can move forward and have control over future situations that are similar to the problems you have encountered in the past. Oftentimes it is how we react to an event or news that dictates how we are going to feel about it, even when we think about it later on.

Spending Time with Unhealthy People

This is especially important when you first start a lifestyle and dietary change. Some of these changes are hard, and if you have someone in your midst who is going to want you to go to McDonald's with them, stay away from them for a while. Surround yourself with others who are interested in changing their health and changing their lifestyle habits. If you can't find anyone locally, you can look for hospital nutrition groups to join. You can also find virtual groups on Twitter or Facebook who may help you stay motivated. Joining my portal will help you track your progress with charts and goal setting, so it can help you stay motivated. Additionally, avoid people who are not supportive of your effort to change your diet and lifestyle habits. If this is someone in the household, then ask them to please give you 60 days of support because you really need it for your health and for your future disease risk.

Toxic Exposure

Exposure to harmful chemicals can trigger inflammation. It is well known that chronic exposure to nicotine and other chemicals found in cigarettes causes significant inflammation in the lungs, eventually leading to lung cancer or chronic bronchitis in many individuals. Exposure to pesticides, aspartame (the artificial sweetener), BPA (found in some plastics), and DES (a drug prescribed for several decades in the mid-twentieth century to prevent miscarriages) has been linked to cancer. Air and traffic pollution have been linked to diabetes, emphysema, and rheumatoid arthritis.[76]

Many cleaning products deliver a fairly large amount of toxicity. I have seen quite a number of janitorial workers struggle with their health. Many of my fibromyalgia patients have been professional cleaners for years. I express my concern to each of them and am able to convince some of them to switch to using less-toxic products that don't risk harm. Some cleaning supplies can irritate the throat and eyes or cause headaches, not to mention what these environmental toxins can do to harm important receptor sites on the surface of cells. Some contain harmful ingredients such as ammonia and bleach. Other products release dangerous fumes, including volatile organic compounds (VOCs). Even natural fragrances such as citrus can produce dangerous pollutants indoors. Research has connected VOCs to respiratory problems, allergic reactions, and headaches.[77] Studies have also connected the chemicals in cleaning supplies to asthma and other respiratory illnesses.[78] Don't mix cleaning products that contain bleach with ones that contain ammonia. Doing so can create harmful effects, including chronic breathing problems and even death.[79]

Products that may contain VOCs and other unhealthy chemicals are listed below:

- aerosol spray products, including health, beauty, and cleaning products
- air fresheners
- chlorine bleach
- detergent and dishwashing liquid
- dry-cleaning chemicals
- furniture and floor polish
- oven cleaners
- rug and upholstery cleaners
- pesticides and herbicides

There are also many food additives that can affect your health significantly. While they may seem harmless, and most are generally recognized as safe by the Food and Drug Administration, some of these food additives can cause significant harm. There is just no reason that we should be consuming food additives and preservatives when we can buy or grow the food fresh and avoid foods that have unwanted chemicals.

The following is a list of common food additives that you should avoid:

- Nitrites and nitrates
  » Found in cured meats such as bacon, hot dogs, sausages, and salami. Nitrates, which come from nitrites, react with proteins to form nitrosamine, a known cancer-causing compound. Nitrites have been mostly linked to stomach cancer.
- Potassium bromate
  » Used in baked goods like bread and cracker dough to strengthen the dough and help it rise during the baking process. It has been shown to cause tumors in animals, can be toxic to the kidneys, and can damage DNA. The United Kingdom, Canada, and the European Union prohibit the use of potassium bromate in food.

- Propyl paraben
  - » Food and Drug Administration considers this compound to be generally recognized as safe (henceforth GRAS).
  - » Disrupts the endocrine system by acting as a weak synthetic estrogen. Has been linked to decreased sperm count, may decrease testosterone levels, and has been shown to alter the expression of genes, especially in breast cancer cells. It is used in tortillas, muffins, and other baked goods.
- Butylated hydroxyanisole (BHA)
  - » GRAS.
  - » Mainly used as a food preservative. National Toxicology Program classifies it as "reasonably anticipated to be a human carcinogen," and the European Union considers it an endocrine disruptor. At higher doses in rats it can lower testosterone, decrease sperm count, and decrease thyroid hormone.
- Butylated hydroxytoluene (BHT)
  - » GRAS.
  - » Chemical cousin to BHA and also used as a food preservative. In rat studies, it has been linked to endocrine disruption, liver tumors, developmental issues, and thyroid changes.
- Propyl gallate
  - » GRAS.
  - » Used as a preservative in edible fats such as sausage or lard. Some old rat studies show endocrine disruption, but there's not enough data to confirm or deny the health risks of propyl gallate. My feeling is that it is still a chemical and still foreign; therefore it should be avoided.
- Theobromide
  - » GRAS.
  - » Found naturally in green tea and chocolate, but now is being used in fourfold larger quantities in breads, cereals, and sports drinks. Theobromide was able to gain GRAS status without the approval from the Food and Drug Administration.
- Flavor ingredients
  - » GRAS.
  - » "Artificial flavor" is very common and finds its way into about

one out of every seven foods. "Natural flavor" is on the list of thousands of foods, accounting for about one-quarter of foods. In order for the "natural flavor" to be successful, flavor mixtures sometimes contain natural or artificial emulsifiers, solvents, and preservatives that are called "incidental additives." Sadly, when a manufacturer uses incidental additives, they are not required to disclose their presence on food labels. Flavoring mixtures added to food are complex and can contain more than 100 distinct substances. The non-flavor chemicals that have other functional properties often make up 80 to 90 percent of the mixture.

- Artificial coloring
  - » GRAS.
  - » Used in cosmetics and foods. Remember that your skin is an excellent absorber, so don't think that if you don't eat it, you won't be exposed to it. Artificial coloring has had conflicting studies on childhood behavior and asthma. The caramel colorings have been linked to cancer-causing chemicals. Avoiding specific artificial colors can be difficult because current regulation allows food manufacturers to simply print "artificial color" on the product label if the ingredient is on an FDA-approved list.
- Diacetyl
  - » GRAS.
  - » Used as a butter flavoring on microwave popcorn, to flavor dairy products such as yogurt and cheese, in "brown flavorings" such as butterscotch and maple, and in fruit flavorings such as strawberry and raspberry. Diacetyl can lead to a severe and irreversible respiratory condition called bronchiolitis obliterans, which leads to inflammation and permanent scarring of the airways, especially in factory workers around the chemical in the preparation of the food.
- Phosphate food additives
  - » Among the most common food additives. It is included in a lot of unhealthy fast food and processed items. Phosphate additives may be harmful to people with kidney disease, and it increases cardiovascular risk.
- Aluminum additives
  - » Aluminum additives have lessened in recent years. Additives

containing aluminum, such as sodium aluminum phosphate and sodium aluminum sulfate, are used as stabilizers in many processed foods, but were once also used as a preservative in many beauty products such as contact solution, eye drops, and other liquid products. Additionally, thimerosal, a mercury preservative, was used heavily in vaccines in the past but hasn't been used in childhood vaccinations since July of 1999.

» Aluminum has been linked to Alzheimer's and neurological defects in the womb if the mother is exposed.[80]

To begin reducing your exposure to harmful chemicals, first consider where your exposure may be coming from. Here are some suggestions:

- If you live in a large city with quite a bit of air pollution, you may be unable to completely avoid exposure. But perhaps you can avoid getting on your bike during rush hour, or at least change your route to choose quiet residential streets rather than heavily-trafficked main thoroughfares where you'll be riding alongside lots of smog-producing cars.
- Avoid drinking tap water at restaurants and other places. Get a filter for your tap water at home to avoid the heavy metals and harmful chemicals found in some water.
- Reduce your exposure to fertilizers and pesticides by finding a park nearby where the maintenance crew doesn't spray. The parks with perfect green lawns most likely are heavily sprayed.
- Avoid ordering animal products at a restaurant unless you know they're organic.
- Avoid arsenic and other harmful chemicals by not smoking.
- Avoid other artificial chemicals by eliminating your intake of processed foods.
- Avoid eating fast food.
- Avoid all microwavable foods.
- Read labels and avoid all food additives and chemicals.
- In your home, one product at a time, gradually get rid of all the chemically laden ones. Use natural cleaners, natural shampoos and soaps, and house paint that doesn't release VOCs. Practice organic gardening and lawn-care methods.

- Avoid using perfumes and lotions that contain artificial chemicals, as well as unnaturally scented candles, air fresheners, and plug-ins.
- Begin the challenging process of getting rid of all your plastic. It's okay to store food in some plastics that are BPA-free, but don't heat food in them. For water bottles, choose stainless steel or BPA-free plastic. Don't use bottled water unless you have to.

Reduce Exposure to Mercury and Other Heavy Metals

Mercury is a large, controversial subject. I believe it is important to speak about because even the Environmental Protection Agency (EPA) believes that overconsumption of mercury negatively affects health. A significant source of mercury contamination for humans is related to fish consumption. Although fish are healthy to eat due to their content of essential fatty acids, some species contain dangerous amounts of mercury. Each variety needs to be considered individually.

The following comes from the EPA/FDA advisory on fish consumption for pregnant and nursing women, women who may become pregnant, and young children:

By following the recommendations below for selecting and eating fish or shellfish, women and young children will receive the benefits of eating fish and shellfish and can be confident that they have reduced their exposure to the harmful effects of mercury.

- Do not eat shark, swordfish, king mackerel, or tilefish because they contain high levels of mercury.
- Eat up to 12 ounces (two average meals) a week of a variety of fish and shellfish that are lower in mercury.
- Five of the most commonly eaten fish that are low in mercury are shrimp, canned light tuna, salmon, pollock, and catfish.
- Check local advisories about the safety of fish caught by family and friends in your local lakes, rivers, and coastal areas. If no advice is available, eat up to 6 ounces (one average meal) per week of fish you catch from local waters,

but don't consume any other fish during that week.[81]

My recommendation regarding the consumption of tuna is to highly limit it. We generally limit our tuna consumption to eating sushi at a restaurant. If we want canned fish, we purchase salmon. Occasionally we have gotten freshly canned salmon from our patients. This is the best choice because we know how long it has been canned.

Mercury used to be prevalent as a preservative in many health and beauty products, such as contact-lens solution. In recent years, companies have reduced or eliminated their use of mercury in consumer products, mostly due to demand. Read labels, and avoid purchasing any product containing thimerosal. As mentioned above, thimerosal was used as a preservative in vaccinations. It has now been removed from most childhood vaccinations. Make sure you educate yourself prior to vaccinating a young infant.

Other heavy metals can be found in many products, including cigarettes, canned products, water, well water, old paint, old pipes, fertilizers, soil, rivers, lakes, pesticides, and more. Visit the EPA's website if you desire more information about the presence of heavy metals in your environment.

Self-Medicating with Substances

Whatever the substance you are using to make yourself feel better, stop. Be it alcohol, sugar, cookies, marijuana, cigarettes, or any other drug, understand that the good feelings provided by these items are temporary and they falsely change your brain neurochemistry, fooling you into thinking you feel good for the moment. But in all actuality, they will leave you more depleted than you were before you used the substance. If you have good willpower, then I suggest quitting cold turkey. Tell 10 people whom you are close to or whom you spend a lot of time with to help you quit. They can help you with reminders and by keeping you busy while you quit.

If you need additional help, ask for it. Seek out the nearest AA or NA meeting or counselor to help you quit your addiction. If it is a food or cigarette addiction, I have seen hypnotherapy be very effective at helping people quit. Whatever the addiction is, most likely you will need help and support, and I suggest working on these issues first before starting this program so that when you enter this program, you enter it with a clear mind. Substances, even foods, cloud the brain neurochemistry and the senses, and can prevent you from succeeding at a healthy diet and lifestyle program.

Overeating

Make sure you eat enough, but make sure you are conscious about overeating. There are many things that stimulate our potential for overeating. We may have an emotional connection with food so that when we eat, we stimulate endorphins and feel better about ourselves. We may eat when we are nervous or stressed about something. We eat socially all the time, and this is definitely when some overeating or wrong food choices can occur. We may just overeat because we crave food and the taste of food. We may overeat because the food tastes so good and we are eating it too fast.

Be mindful of your habits over this next 60 days and beyond. I ask my patients to try to stop eating when they are 70 percent full. This can some-times be hard, but if you begin the habit of stopping there, then for the 30 minutes after your meal, you usually find that you are completely full, and then you just saved yourself the extra calories that you would have eaten if you had continued to eat when you wanted to. Sometimes stopping when 70 percent full and then setting a timer for 10–15 minutes later helps you manage the need for an extra serving. If you are still hungry or wanting the extra serving 15 minutes later, then maybe you are still a bit hungry, but keep the next serving very small. Most of the time, after 15 minutes goes by, you feel fine and you don't need or want the extra serving.

Sometimes I feel a little hungry or want a sweet, but I know that I ate an hour ago and that my hunger is mostly emotional. When this happens, I have to get creative to keep myself from reaching into the refrigerator, mostly because I know I shouldn't be hungry, so I have to figure out how not to eat. This may be something that you struggle with, too.

Tricks to Help You Stop Overeating

As you can see, there are many reasons that people overeat. There's no specific way to stop overeating that works for every person, but rather there are many different ways to help your body learn not to eat too much. Some may work better for you than others. Below is a list of six tricks you can try to help you quell your overeating:

1. Only fill your plate with how much you should eat, and then put the rest of the food away before you start eating. This helps you limit what you are eating to only one serving and keeps the temptation of eating more at bay. If this doesn't work, then only make enough for that one serving so there is no extra left over.
2. Don't wait too long between meals, because when you are really hungry, you will be in urgent need of balancing your blood sugar levels and then you will seek out unhealthy foods, or you may end up binging on foods rather then preparing yourself a meal.
3. Eat breakfast.
4. Pour a 20-ounce glass of water and take small sips until it is finished. I often feel very full after this and then no longer want to eat. I have experimented with putting various things into the water to satisfy my craving. Here are some ideas of what to put in the water for some flavoring:

    a. Slices of cucumber
    b. Raspberries
    c. Juice from lemon
    d. Lemon wedges
    e. Lime wedges
    f. Apple cider vinegar
    g. Mint leaves
    h   Basil leaves
    i. Drink plain sparkling water (no sweetener or flavoring)

5. If I have just finished a meal but feel like I want something

more or feel like I want something sweet, I will set a timer for 15–20 minutes. If I am still hungry when the timer goes off, then I allow myself something additional such as a few nuts or seeds.

6. If I am feeling full just after a meal but still want to eat because I am not feeling satisfied, then I will drink a small amount of water, such as two to four ounces, and then brush my teeth. Brushing your teeth will oftentimes curb the cravings you have for something sweet after a meal.

Chart of Habits to Avoid and Include

Avoid	Include
Watching TV	Sleep—over seven hours nightly
Negative thinking	Exercise daily or at least five times per week
Spending time with unhealthy people	Meditation or stress relief daily
Toxic exposure	Positive affirmations daily
Self-medicating with substances	Filtered water—half your weight in ounces daily
Overeating	Chewing your food well
Drinking while eating	A ritual for eating
	Family meals when you can
	Eating breakfast
	Snacks

CHAPTER 12

The Supplement Program

Breakfast or Lunch Supplements

- Freedom supplement
- Vitamin C: 1,000 mg
- Chromium: 200 mcg

Between Meals

Best in place of the midmorning snack. Fiber supplement: pick one of the following in either capsules or powder. Make sure that if you are taking capsules you take them with enough water. I suggest 12 ounces of water whether you take the supplement in powder or capsule form.

- Inulin: 5 grams in water or taken with 12 ounces of water
- Psyllium husk powder (plantago asiatica, seed): 1.5 grams in water or taken with 12 ounces of water

Lunch or Dinner Supplements

- Freedom supplement
- Vitamin C: 1,000 mg
- Chromium: 200 mcg

Supplements	A.M.	Between Meals	P.M.
Glucose Freedom	4 capsules	Fiber and 12 oz. of filtered water	4 capsules
Vitamin C	1,000 mg		1,000 mg
Chromium	200 mcg		200 mcg

CHAPTER 13

Getting Prepared in the Kitchen

I can guarantee that if we take anyone who can chew vegetables and have them eat eight cups of vegetables per day for a few weeks we will see improvement of some sort. The main problem I encounter when people start doing this is that their digestion is sometimes not ready for it, and they can feel awfully gassy when they first begin. The simple solution is to steam all the vegetables at first so that you are able to digest them better. I am going to offer some very easy suggestions to help you understand that cooking can be rather quick and easy, especially with simple ingredients.

Be Prepared and Don't Be Afraid

Taking lunches and snacks along with you when you leave the house prevents you from getting lost in the American wasteland of fast food if you become urgently hungry. Resisting the temptations of sweets and treats at work takes willpower and backbone. Understanding creates willpower: understanding the risks involved when making poor food choices, understanding the risk inflammation and blood sugar elevations pose to your long-term health, and understanding how great it feels to enjoy vibrant health and well-being.

Know that with any change, you are bound to make mistakes! Don't be afraid to fail. Behind every success often lies a significant number of failures. Be creative. Don't think you have to follow the recipes or the lifestyle plan verbatim. Make it your own thing. Create your own meals from the ideas presented in this book, and learn to season foods in your own unique way. Experiment a lot! Your experiments may result in the occasional funny moment in your kitchen or at the dinner table with your family, but they will also force you to learn and improve your skills.

Navigating Food Choices

Food is prepared in many ways. Sometimes the method of food preparation can interfere with the food's quality and nutrient content. Below are my suggestions for choosing foods that are as natural and nutrient-dense as possible. The main goal here is to get back to our roots. That means greatly reducing or eliminating consumption of artificial additives, chemicals, preservatives, and unnatural substances, many of which have been linked to cancer and other illnesses.

- **Filter your drinking and cooking water.** Consider this a golden rule in your kitchen and for your family. Plain tap water simply contains too many chemicals that can affect your health, such as heavy metals, hormones, residues from chemicals used in treatment facilities, and farming chemicals. Furthermore, the balance of minerals in your water may be off. A filter can help remove unwanted chemicals and correct imbalances. Many different types of water filters are available; spend some time researching them before purchasing one. You can begin with a simple system, like a Brita pitcher, which utilizes a carbon filter, but for the long term, consider going with a more advanced filtration system for your entire home.
- **Organic meat is best.** Organic meat is free of toxic chemicals. If you can't find organic meat, then look for hormone-free meat. Organic meat usually comes from animals that have been grass fed or, in the case of poultry, have been given feed free of additives such as antibiotics. Grass-fed animal proteins are better than proteins from

grain-fed animals. Cattle and buffalo were meant to graze on grass, and that is what they do for most of their lives. Most commercially raised cattle will graze on grass but will be finished off in the last months of their lives with grains such as corn to increase their weight and fat content. The meat taste we have grown to love as Americans comes from this extra fat content. Grass-fed animals are leaner; they have one-third to one-half the fat of grain-fed animals of the same size. The meat from grass-fed animals is higher in good nutrients: beef from a grass-fed cow has three times the vitamin E content and is higher in omega-3 fatty acids, providing a better omega-3 to omega-6 ratio than beef from a grain-fed cow. Grass-fed beef also has a higher content of conjugated linoleic acid (CLA), a lesser-known but important group of polyunsaturated fatty acids found in beef, lamb, and dairy products. The less our farming practices adhere to an animal's natural growth and development patterns, the greater the risk of something going wrong, such as the meat being contaminated or the animal getting sick. It is also important to avoid meat from animals that have been fed antibiotics or hormones or have spent time around pesticides. Hormones fed to animals are used to increase their growth, but they are detrimental to health. Many of the common cancers, such as prostate, breast, and ovarian cancers, are often directly related to excess hormone influence.

- **Whenever possible, choose organic vegetables and fruits.** Produce is best purchased fresh and local. A few vegetables and fruits, such as peas and berries, may be purchased frozen for ease of use. Never buy canned vegetables and fruits, with the exception of canned tomatoes on rare occasions. If you are on a tight budget and organic produce seems out of reach cost-wise, be aware that there are a few fruits and vegetables that are more important to purchase organic because they are heavily sprayed with chemicals when grown following conventional methods. A comprehensive list of both the cleanest and the most contaminated fruits and vegetables can be found at the website of the Environmental Working Group: www. ewg.org/foodnews/summary.

- **Use Real Salt over other types of sea salt or table salt.** Many table salts contain added anticaking agents or dextrose, which is a potato sugar. Other types of sea salt are sometimes more processed and may not offer the variety of minerals that Real Salt does. Real Salt brand sea salt comes from Redmond, Utah, and has a distinct, rich taste. Its off-white color comes from the many trace minerals (as many as 60 different ones) that are present in the salt. Himalayan or Celtic salts are also acceptable, but I prefer using a salt local to our area rather than from other parts of the world.

- **Buy fresh foods over canned.** Exceptions to this guideline include coconut milk, canned wild-caught salmon, and beans (occasionally) when you are in a pinch and haven't soaked any.

- **Purchase wild-caught fish instead of farm-raised.** Wild fish contains significantly higher levels of omega-3 fatty acids, the important fats that help our bodies ward off cancer and other inflammatory illnesses. They are also extremely important in supporting brain function and helping maintain memory and cognitive ability into older age. Farmed fish such as salmon often contains dyes to make it appear rich in omega-3 fatty acids.

- **Avoid processed foods as much as possible.** Chips, boxed foods, prepared meals, cold cuts, hot dogs, frozen pizzas, frozen snacks, SpaghettiOs, and prepared macaroni and cheese are just some examples of processed foods that should be avoided.

Food Items to Keep on Hand/Shopping List

Below is a list of some helpful items to keep in your kitchen. Having these groceries on hand can minimize your trips to the store when you're planning a meal and will make it easier to throw together healthy dinners spontaneously. A meal of beans and rice is an easy staple you can prepare in a pinch, even if you haven't been able to go grocery shopping.

- dried grains and legumes: quinoa, lentils, white beans, garbanzo beans
- canned goods: salmon, beans, coconut milk
- dried spices and herbs: cinnamon, ginger, basil, garlic powder, onion powder, mustard powder, cumin, turmeric, nutmeg, peppercorns or fresh-ground pepper, Real Salt
- dried goods: unsweetened coconut, sunflower seeds, pumpkin seeds, hemp seeds, chia seeds, flax seeds
- fresh vegetables in season, including salad greens
- fresh berries
- frozen goods: homemade broths, berries for smoothies
- condiments: gluten-free tamari sauce, mustard with no added sugar, homemade mayonnaise
- vinegars: apple cider vinegar, red wine vinegar, white vinegar, others as desired
- fresh herbs and spices: garlic, onions, ginger, parsley
- fats and oils: organic butter, coconut oil, olive oil
- milk and eggs: unsweetened almond milk, unsweetened hemp milk, organic eggs
- specifics for the recipes you want to prepare during the week

Making Healthy Eating Easier

It is important to reduce kitchen time and make your kitchen and yourself more efficient. This task is not always easy, especially with our busy lifestyles involving work, kids in sports, and other commitments. Here are a few tips for reducing kitchen time:

Food Preparation

- Pre-chop vegetables you know you will be using during the week.
- Pre-chop garlic and onions, and keep them refrigerated in airtight containers for use.
- Prepare everything for dinner when you are making lunch so that dinner is much easier to get on the table.
- Make stocks and broths ahead of time, and store them in small quantities in the freezer.
- Make large batches of soup so you have extra to freeze for a later date.
- Prepare extra servings when you're cooking dinner so you have leftovers for lunch the next day.
- Do not microwave food. If you microwave at all, do so sparingly because the process destroys important nutrients.

Food Equipment

- Small food chopper.
- Coffee grinder (for grinding nuts and seeds).
- Blender or Vitamix. A Vitamix is an extremely high-powered blender that can handle a full range of tasks, from making a smoothie, to grinding nuts and seeds, to making your own flours. If you have a Vitamix, then you generally won't need a coffee grinder or food chopper.
- Food processor. Superior to the Vitamix for grating a large quantity of ingredients such as zucchini and other vegetables, especially if you don't want your vegetables

to be blended too fine.
- Nonaluminum sauté pans and ovenware.
- Parchment paper. Parchment paper has saved me hundreds of hours of cleaning pans. You can line any baking pan with parchment paper for a nearly hassle-free cleanup.

Cooking Tips

- Use easy steaming procedures for simple vegetable side dishes topped with a small amount of your favorite sauce. You can use an inexpensive basket-style steamer, or just put half an inch of filtered water in a saucepan, add your chopped vegetables, and cook over medium heat. With either method, steam until the vegetables have a bright color but are still crunchy-tender. You may need to add more water if it evaporates during steaming. You can also save the water that you steamed your vegetables in and add it to a smoothie or cook lentils in it so that you obtain the nutrients in the water.
- Learn to improvise! Don't think you always need a recipe. The more you cook, the more you will learn to guess what you need, and the more you will learn about how seasonings blend together. You'll get better at substituting when you don't have the exact ingredient. Don't be afraid to experiment with new ingredients.
- Make extra servings of lentils or beans when preparing a meal, and freeze the extra in airtight containers. It is handy to be able to pull out some frozen lentils and add to a salad or other meal for additional protein.
- Eat raw one night per week. This can be an easy meal of cut-up veggies, fruits, and dips. Often, we will throw veggies and fruit into the blender with water and have a green drink for the evening. This feels very refreshing and healthy. Make sure you are able to tolerate raw foods before incorporating "Raw Night" into your household.

Organization and Preparation

- Keep your pantry, refrigerator, and spice area well organized.
- Make lists when you run out of items that you need from the store.
- Plan meals before you grocery shop.
- Have "go-to" meals that are easy and quick but still nutritious and healthy. This helps to reduce unhealthy snacking.
- Have ideas for healthy snacks, and avoid buying snacks that you will feel guilty about eating.
- Clean the kitchen as you prepare meals. Utilize the natural gaps in time that occur when cooking to wash the dishes and utensils you have used and no longer need. That way, many of your dishes are already rinsed and placed in the dishwasher before your meal is ready to eat.
- Pack your lunches, and take snacks with you everywhere you go. Don't rely on finding food while you're out. Most of the time you won't be able to find much that's healthy. Carrying snacks will also keep you and your children happier by avoiding blood sugar crashes and the resulting moodiness.

Food Attitude

- Have fun when you go shopping. Take the whole family so that you all participate in choosing foods. Think about foods and cooking in a new perspective. Don't fight the change; accept and appreciate it for what it will bring to you and your family.
- Get the children involved. Have them pick out a new vegetable at the store, and then go home and research how to cook it.
- Grow a garden so that you have control over what you grow and can enjoy eating from the crop you harvest. Even if you don't have garden space, many plants can be grown on a sunny patio.

Measurement Conversions

Liquid Measures

- 1 cup = 8 fluid ounces = 250 milliliters = 16 tablespoons
- 1 tablespoon = 1/2 fluid ounce = 16 milliliters = 3 teaspoons
- 1 teaspoon = 1/6 fluid ounce = 5 1/3 milliliters

Egg Sizes (Large Is the US Standard for Cooking)

- 1 egg = 1.5 fluid ounces = 1.75 ounces without shell = 50 grams without shell
- 1 egg white = 2 tablespoons = 32 milliliters = 30 grams
- 1 egg yolk = 1 tablespoon = 16 milliliters = 20 grams

Solid Fats (Butter, Coconut Oil)

- 8 tablespoons = 4 ounces = 1/4 pound = 115 grams = 1 stick (butter)

Temperatures

- 250°F = 120°C = very low
- 300°F = 150°C = low
- 325°F = 165°C = moderately low
- 350°F = 180°C = moderate
- 375°F = 190°C = moderately hot
- 400°F = 200°C = hot
- 450°F = 230°C = very hot
- 500°F = 260°C = extremely hot; most broilers are set at this temperature or above

CHAPTER 14

Sample Freedom Diet Recipes

Your diet will consist of a breakfast, lunch, and dinner schedule with snacks in between. You will need to wrap your head around eating vegetables for breakfast. I am not sure why we have omitted this important nutrient from one of our most important meals. The suggestions are listed below, with the recipes following.

Breakfast:

Poached egg over arugula topped with avocado and salsa
Steamed kale served with seasoned ground turkey
Hard- or soft-boiled egg served with light green salad
Chia seed pudding with berries

Lunch:

Spinach salad with steamed chicken, yam, and goat cheese
Strawberry green salad with pumpkin seeds
Arugula and hummus with warmed ground beef
Quinoa tabouli with parsley lamb patty

Dinner:

Steamed green beans with salmon
Taco salad
Rosemary roasted vegetables with green lentils
Green chicken chili

Beverages:

Green smoothie
Green drink
Protein fiber blender drink
Homemade almond milk

Snacks:

Raw sunflower seeds
Raw pumpkin seeds
Protein Delight seed crackers
Hummus
Celery with hummus
Berries
Raw cucumbers, carrots, peppers, and other vegetables
    on the okay list

Poached Egg over Arugula Topped with Avocado and Salsa

Per serving: 200 calories — 8.9 g protein — 9.4 g carbohydrate — 5.6 g fiber — 15.3 g total fat — 3.0 g saturated fat — 186.0 mg cholesterol — 310.0 mg sodium

1 egg
4 cups water
1 tablespoon vinegar
1 ½ cups arugula
½ avocado
Salsa to taste, no sugar added

To poach eggs: Heat water and vinegar to simmering in medium saucepan or skillet. Crack egg and gently add to water. Simmer very gently until whites are set and yolk is still somewhat soft, about 3 minutes.

Prepare arugula in a meal-sized bowl, gently place poached egg over the greens, and top with the avocado and salsa. You may lightly salt and pepper the dish if desired.

Serve warm.

SERVES 1.

Recipe Tidbit:

Poaching is an art. If you don't get it right the first time, try it again. I learned how to poach eggs when my kitchen was being remodeled and I only had a hot plate and a toaster oven. I was missing eggs and decided to try poaching them. I found that I loved them as an easy preparation over the months my kitchen was in disarray. Additionally, poaching is the healthiest way to prepare an egg. Alter this recipe by swapping out the greens for another kind or adding condiments of your choice. Double and triple this recipe if you have guests. It is easy to poach more than one egg at a time in the same simmering water.

Steamed Kale Served with Seasoned Ground Turkey

PER SERVING: 372 CALORIES — 27.6 G PROTEIN — 15.7 G
CARBOHYDRATE — 5.8 G FIBER — 24.5 G TOTAL FAT — 14.4 G
SATURATED FAT — 83.9 MG CHOLESTEROL — 419.7 MG SODIUM

2 tablespoons coconut oil
1 red onion, minced
3 cloves garlic, minced
8 cups kale, stems removed and chopped fine
¼ cup water
1 pound ground turkey
½ teaspoon salt
2 tablespoons coconut oil
½ teaspoon pepper
½ teaspoon thyme
½ teaspoon curry
½ teaspoon cumin
½ teaspoon turmeric
1 pint cherry tomatoes (optional)

In a medium-sized saucepan over medium heat, sauté garlic and onion in 2 table-spoons of coconut oil or butter. While the onions and garlic are cooking, in a separate saucepan combine the kale and water, cover, and turn on low heat for 2 minutes. Then turn off the heat, remove the pan from the heat, and set aside, still covered. When the onions become translucent in the other pan, add the ground turkey and seasonings and cook until the meat is no longer pink, about 7–10 minutes. Finally, add the cherry tomatoes, stir to combine, and remove from heat.

Divide the kale into three separate bowls and top with a third of the turkey mixture. Mustard, spices, or flavorful condiments can be used atop this mixture as long as they have no added sugar or artificial sweetener.

Serve warm.

SERVES 4.

Recipe Tidbit:

If you are cooking only for yourself, then use the entire pound of turkey but only prepare 2 cups of the steamed kale. You can reserve the remaining turkey for lettuce wraps or warm it up and serve it over a salad for lunch. You can also add the turkey to a soup.

Hard- or Soft-Boiled Egg Served over Light Green Salad

PER SERVING: 410 CALORIES — 15.1 G PROTEIN — 10.8 G CARBOHYDRATE — 4.7 G FIBER — 35.7 G TOTAL FAT — 4.9 G SATURATED FAT — 186.5 MG CHOLESTEROL — 134.4 MG SODIUM

1 egg, hard- or soft-boiled
2 cups mixed salad greens
¼ cup sunflower seeds

For the dressing:
1 cup red wine vinegar
¾ cup olive oil
1 tablespoon dried basil
¼ teaspoon salt
¼ teaspoon pepper
1 tablespoon mustard

To hard-boil eggs: Place the egg(s) in a large saucepan and cover with room-temperature water, filling the pan to at least 1–2 inches above the top of the egg(s). Bring the water to boil over medium to high heat. Once the water is boiling, cover with a lid and remove from heat. Allow time for the eggs to continue cooking, about 10 minutes. If you want to eat immediately, place in a colander and rinse with cold water. Peel and serve. Otherwise, transfer the eggs to the refrigerator for future use.

To soft-boil eggs: Place the egg(s) in a large saucepan and cover with room temperature water, filling the pan to at least 1–2 inches above the top of the egg(s). Bring the water to boil over medium to high heat. Once the water is boiling, cover with a lid and remove from heat. Allow the eggs to sit for 1–2 minutes. Transfer them to a large colander and rinse with cold water to stop further cooking. Peel and serve. Transfer to the refrigerator if you will be using them at a later time.

Place salad greens and sunflower seeds in a bowl. Combine the dressing ingredients, and toss about 2 tablespoons of dressing gently with salad greens. Top with a hard- or soft-boiled egg.

SERVES 1.

Recipe Tidbit:

Soft-boiled eggs are generally a little healthier for you. If you are going to be preparing this breakfast with a soft-boiled egg, then I suggest you soft-boil the egg when you want to eat the meal. If you are going to be using hard-boiled eggs, it is okay to make them at the time you want the meal and eat them warm, or you can make them ahead of time and eat the salad and egg cold. Making them ahead of time can save you a lot of time in the morning.

Chia Seed Pudding with Berries

PER SERVING: 435 CALORIES — 7.6 G PROTEIN — 21.1 G CAR-
BOHYDRATE — 13.2 G FIBER — 38.2 G TOTAL FAT — 26.2 G
SATURATED FAT — 0.0 MG CHOLESTEROL — 228.8 MG SODIUM

½ cup chia seeds
1 cup full-fat coconut milk
1 cup unsweetened almond milk
1 teaspoon vanilla extract
½ teaspoon cinnamon
½ teaspoon cardamom
Very small pinch salt
Fresh raspberries, blueberries, or blackberries

*Whisk all ingredients except berries together for at least 5 minutes and pour
into a large serving glass. Cover and store in refrigerator until set, about
half an hour. Longer sitting time is also fine. Serve chilled and topped with
berries.*

SERVES 2.

Recipe Tidbit:

Avoiding most sugar items for this diet can be a bit trying at first,
but the longer you are sugar free, the more you will appreciate the
natural sweetness of berries and vegetables. Remember to also avoid
all artificial sweeteners as they can interrupt your body's natural
sugar-balancing biochemistry. Stevia, which comes from a plant, is the
only sweetener that you are allowed to use for this diet. I always start
with small amounts and increase from there to add sweetness because
using too much stevia can give your food a bitter/astringent taste.

Wilted Spinach Salad with Chicken, Yam, and Goat Cheese

PER SERVING: 419 CALORIES — 42.8 G PROTEIN — 26.9 G CARBOHYDRATE — 4.9 G FIBER — 15.1 G TOTAL FAT — 6.1 G SATURATED FAT — 129.9 MG CHOLESTEROL — 174.6 MG SODIUM

1 pound chicken breast
2 large yams
6 cups spinach
6 tablespoons goat or sheep cheese (omit if dairy intolerant)

For the dressing:
1 clove garlic, minced
¼ cup apple cider vinegar
⅓ cup olive oil
2 tablespoons fresh lemon juice
Salt and pepper to taste

Preheat the oven to 400 degrees Farenheight. Wrap a full yam in tinfoil and place in the oven. Bake for 40 minutes or until the yam is tender. (You can do this step ahead of time if needed.) At the same time, place chicken breasts in baking pan and add filtered water to cover at least the lower half of the chicken breasts. Cover and place in the oven. Bake for about 20 minutes, or until the chicken breasts are white on the inside but still tender. Remove from the oven and allow to cool slightly.

Prepare spinach leaves in a bowl. Cut the chicken into chunks and, for each serving, place 1/3 over 2 cups of spinach leaves, allowing them to wilt slightly. Cut the yam into chunks and place about 1/3 over the chicken and spinach. Top with 2 tablespoons of salad dressing and enjoy.

SERVES 3.

Recipe Tidbit:

Making foods ahead really saves time. For example, we are using chicken breasts and yams in this recipe. If you cook extra chicken, then afterwards you can simply chunk it and make it into chicken salad to be used at an additional meal. If you cook 2-3 yams, you can use them at a later meal, as a snack, or you can chunk them and freeze them to be used in the future. These time-saving tricks can help you adhere to this diet a little better. Come up with as many time-saving tricks as you can throughout the week. After a while, they will become habit, and your preparedness for meals and snacks will improve. You also can double or triple this recipe.

Strawberry Green Salad with Pumpkin Seeds

Per serving: 456 calories — 19.8 g protein — 24.1 g carbohydrate — 8.3 g fiber — 35.4 g total fat — 5.9 g saturated fat — 0.0 mg cholesterol — 109.3 mg sodium

2 cups mixed greens
1 cup strawberries, stems removed, cut into halves
¼ cup pumpkin seeds

For the dressing:
1 clove garlic
¼ onion
¼ cup olive oil
¼ cup balsamic vinegar
1 tablespoon mustard
¼ cup strawberries
¼ teaspoon salt
¼ teaspoon pepper
1 tablespoon organic feta cheese (optional)
1 heaping tablespoon pumpkin seeds

To make the dressing, grind the 1 tablespoon of pumpkin seeds in a high-powered blender or coffee grinder. Add all other dressing ingredients and blend until smooth. Refrigerate until use.

Combine greens, strawberries, and pumpkin seeds in a bowl. Top with 2 tablespoons of dressing and serve chilled.

SERVES 1.

Recipe Tidbit:

Nuts and seeds are best if they are eaten raw. You can enjoy some of your nuts roasted but most should be enjoyed raw. You can even soak the nuts or seeds ahead of time to make them easier to digest. An overnight soak is easiest. Save the rest of this dressing to be used in other salads.

Arugula and Hummus with Warmed Ground Beef

PER SERVING: 584 CALORIES — 32.0 G PROTEIN — 21.0 G CAR-
BOHYDRATE — 4.8 G FIBER — 42.3 G TOTAL FAT — 14.1 G
SATURATED FAT — 99.8 MG CHOLESTEROL — 540.3 MG SODIUM

2 tablespoons olive oil
3 cloves garlic, minced
1 onion, minced
1 pound ground beef, organic and grass fed
⅓ teaspoon salt
¼ teaspoon pepper
1 teaspoon chili powder
1 teaspoon turmeric powder
1 teaspoon paprika
1 teaspoon garlic powder
1 teaspoon onion powder
¼ teaspoon cayenne pepper
6 cups arugula
¾ cup hummus

Sauté the garlic and onion in the olive oil over medium heat. After the
onions and garlic are translucent, about 3–5 minutes, add the ground beef,
salt, pepper, and seasonings and cook until the meat is thoroughly cooked,
about 7–10 minutes.

Arrange the arugula on a large dinner plate. Top with the hummus.
Spoon the ground beef mixture over the hummus and serve immediately.

SERVES 3.

Recipe Tidbit:

This is a great, flavorful meat to use for taco salads. You can thinly
slice jicama into "taco shells" for making tacos. Grass-fed ground beef
is a great occasional source of protein. Make sure to always balance the
ground beef with plenty of vegetables. Remember that consuming a

lot of vegetables alongside your protein will help to maintain balanced blood sugar levels.

Quinoa Tabouli

PER SERVING: 654 CALORIES — 20.2 G PROTEIN — 37.1 G CARBOHYDRATE — 7.8 G FIBER — 47.2 G TOTAL FAT — 6.1 G SATURATED FAT — 0.0 MG CHOLESTEROL — 592.2 MG SODIUM

1 cup uncooked quinoa
2 cups water
1 bunch parsley, stems removed, and chopped fine
1 cup hemp hearts
1 cup tomatoes, chopped
¾ cup lemon juice
½ cup olive oil
3 cloves garlic, minced
3 tablespoons minced mint leaves
1 teaspoon salt

Heat water and quinoa to boiling in a medium saucepan. Reduce the heat and simmer, covered, until water is absorbed, about 15 minutes. Place parsley in a large glass bowl. Spoon the hot quinoa over the parsley, cover and set aside for about 10 minutes. Transfer to refrigerator to chill. After the parsley and quinoa are chilled, add remaining ingredients and serve chilled. Top with hummus if desired or pour over additional salad greens.

SERVES 4.

Recipe Tidbit:

I love tabouli and this is my favorite version. The quinoa offers a complete protein. Mint helps ease and promote digestion and can help to relieve bloating and gas. Even the aroma of mint is known to activate the salivary glands, and other glands that secrete digestive enzymes, thereby facilitating digestion. This explains its long history of use in the culinary arts.

Parsley Lamb Patty

PER SERVING: 304 CALORIES — 27.8 G PROTEIN — 2.2 G CARBOHYDRATE — 0.7 G FIBER — 20.1 G TOTAL FAT — 7.6 G SATURATED FAT — 103.8 MG CHOLESTEROL — 362.3 MG SODIUM

1 pound ground lamb
1 pound ground turkey
3 cloves garlic, minced
½ onion, minced
¾ teaspoon salt
1 teaspoon pepper
¼ teaspoon cayenne
½ teaspoon allspice powder
1 teaspoon cumin
½ teaspoon cinnamon
¼ cup parsley, stems removed, minced
3 large mint leaves, minced

Line two baking pans with parchment paper. Combine all spices with garlic and onion, then combine the spices with the meats. Once the mixture is uniformly mixed, form into 12 balls. Fill each baking pan with 6 balls and lightly press into patties. Cover and put the baking sheets into the refrigerator for at least 1 hour to allow flavors to mingle. Overnight is better. When ready, preheat oven to 375 degrees. Bake until cooked through, about 22–27 minutes.

SERVES 6.

Recipe Tidbit:

I love these little burgers. I like them a little bit spicier so I add another ¼ teaspoon of cayenne.

Steamed Green Beans with Salmon

PER SERVING: 250 CALORIES — 34.4 G PROTEIN — 1.8 G
CARBOHYDRATE — 0.4 G FIBER — 9.0 G TOTAL FAT — 1.6 G SAT-
URATED FAT — 69.6 MG CHOLESTEROL — 380.0 MG SODIUM

1 pound salmon
1 pound green beans, washed and trimmed
Filtered water

Marinade for the salmon:
2 tablespoons mayonnaise
2 tablespoons gluten-free tamari
2 tablespoons olive oil
2 cloves garlic, minced
2 shallots, minced
2 teaspoons ginger, grated
1 teaspoon dill

Seasoning mixture for the beans:
½ teaspoon salt
1 teaspoon garlic powder
1 teaspoon onion powder
½ teaspoon thyme
½ teaspoon basil
1 teaspoon fresh chives, chopped

Begin by combining marinade ingredients in a gallon resealable plastic bag. Place the salmon fillet into the bag and place in the refrigerator for at least 12 hours. Overnight is easiest.

Preheat oven to 350 degrees. Bake salmon, skin side down, covered, for about 12 minutes; uncover and bake for another 3–5 minutes until salmon is tender on the inside but no longer raw-pink.

While the salmon is baking, combine seasoning mixture for the beans. Place green beans in steamer or large pot with half an inch of water on the bottom. Steam the green beans until they are bright green but still crunchy, about 5–7 minutes. Remove from water or steamer, mix with the seasoning mixture, and top with salmon.

SERVES 3.

Recipe Tidbit:

When your beans come out of the steamer, if they are still wet enough, they should combine well with the seasoning mixture. If the mixture seems too dry for the beans, add a little water or melted unsalted organic butter or coconut oil to help combine.

Taco Salad

PER SERVING: 362 CALORIES — 23.6 G PROTEIN — 10.5 G CAR-
BOHYDRATE — 3.9 G FIBER — 25.6 G TOTAL FAT — 13.7 G
SATURATED FAT — 79.4 MG CHOLESTEROL — 395.8 MG SODIUM

2 tablespoons coconut oil
1 onion, minced
3 garlic cloves, minced
½ large green pepper, sliced
½ large red pepper, sliced
½ large yellow pepper, sliced
1 teaspoon paprika
1 teaspoon chili powder
½ teaspoon cumin
½ teaspoon salt
½ teaspoon pepper
¼ teaspoon cayenne
1 pound ground bison, grass fed
8 cups romaine,
washed and chopped
¼ cup chives, chopped
Red or green salsa to taste
Full-fat organic sour cream or yogurt to taste (optional)

Sauté the onions and garlic with the coconut oil in a large sauté pan until translucent, about 3–5 minutes. Add peppers and spices and sauté for another 3 minutes, then remove from heat. In a separate pan, cook the bison over medium heat until there is only a little pink left. Transfer the bison to the pepper and onion mixture, turn the heat to medium, and heat until combined. Cover and turn off the heat.

Meanwhile, divide the romaine between 4 large bowls. Top with bison–pepper mixture and chives. Add salsa and sour cream to taste. Omit the sour cream if you are dairy intolerant or following an anti-inflammatory diet.

SERVES 4.

Recipe Tidbit:

You can do a lot of different things with this taco meat if you have some left over and don't want another salad. Try combining it with an omelet or scrambled eggs and serve over wilted spinach. You can also simply warm it up and wrap it in butter leaf lettuce as a lettuce wrap.

Rosemary Roasted Vegetables with Green Lentils

PER SERVING: 540 CALORIES — 28.8 G PROTEIN — 57.3 G CAR-
BOHYDRATE — 14.2 G FIBER — 24.4 G TOTAL FAT — 3.9 G
SATURATED FAT — 0.0 MG CHOLESTEROL — 1574.7 MG SODIUM

3 ½ cups chicken broth
½ cup green lentils
2 broccoli crowns, chopped
½ small head cauliflower, chopped
2 large carrots, julienned in ½-inch pieces
3 tablespoons olive oil
1 teaspoon balsamic vinegar
1 ½ teaspoon rosemary, minced
Small pinch salt
½ teaspoon pepper
1 teaspoon garlic powder
1 tighly packed cup spinach, stems removed, chopped

Combine the chicken broth and lentils in a small saucepan and heat over medium-high heat until the chicken broth is boiling, then reduce the heat to medium, cover, and cook until the lentils have absorbed all of the chicken broth, about 30 minutes.

While the lentils are cooking, preheat oven to 400 degrees. Place all of the prepared vegetables other than the spinach into a large resealable plastic bag. Add the olive oil, vinegar, rosemary, salt, pepper, and garlic powder, reseal the bag, and then agitate until the vegetables are covered with marinade. Transfer to a large baking pan and bake until the vegetables become bright in color and are softer but still crunchy, about 20 minutes.

Remove the vegetables from the oven, combine with the chopped spinach, and toss the mixture together to combine before serving. Serve immediately.

SERVES 2.

Recipe Tidbit:

You can experiment with various vegetables and can try other lentils for this recipe. Lentils are my favorite legume. They don't have to be soaked, so they are easy to prepare quickly. Even if my cupboards are relatively empty, I can usually make something tasty with lentils and chicken broth or vegetable broth in a very short amount of time. You can dilute the broth to half strength with water; this will help the liquid absorb into the lentils more easily for faster cooking time. Lentils are high in iron, amino acids, and B vitamins. They help to stabilize blood sugar and have been shown to improve cholesterol levels.

Green Chicken Chili

PER SERVING: 248 CALORIES — 19.6 G PROTEIN — 22.0 G
CARBOHYDRATE — 5.1 G FIBER — 9.2 G TOTAL FAT — 1.6 G SATU-
RATED FAT — 40.8 MG CHOLESTEROL — 1138.1 MG SODIUM

1 pound chicken
2 cups filtered water
2 tablespoons olive oil
1 onion, minced
4 cloves garlic, minced
1 ½ salt
2 teaspoons chili poder
1 teaspoon cumin powder
½ teaspoon dried oregano
½ teaspoon cloves, powdered
3 large celery stalks, finely chopped
1 16-oz jar of green salsa, no sweetener added
4 Anaheim chilies, roasted, skins and seeds removed, and chopped
1 12-oz can white beans
1 bunch chard, stems removed, chopped

In a slow cooker, combine water and chicken and cook on high heat for 3 hours. After the chicken is cooked, take it out and place it on a cutting board. Use two forks to tease the chicken into shreds, and set aside. In a large saucepan, sauté the onion and garlic in the olive oil over medium heat until they are translucent. Add the salt, chili powder, cumin, oregano, cloves, and celery and sauté for about 3 more minutes. Add the shredded chicken, salsa, chilies, beans, and chard and heat until just combined and warm. Serve immediately.

SERVES 6.

Recipe Tidbit:

To roast the chilies, start by preheating the broiler. Place the chilies on a large baking pan lined with tinfoil or parchment paper. Place under the broiler for about 10 minutes. The skins will start to look black, forming AGEs. This is okay because we are going to remove the burnt skin. Remove the peppers from the oven and transfer them to a brown paper sack or large resealable plastic bag and close. Allow the peppers to cool slightly in the bag. Remove them from the bag, cut them lengthwise, cut off the top, scoop out the seeds, and chop.

Green Smoothie

PER SERVING: 58 CALORIES — 3.1 G PROTEIN — 12.9
G CARBOHYDRATE — 3.4 G FIBER — 0.6 G TOTAL FAT
— 0.1 G SATURATED FAT — 0.0 MG CHOLESTEROL — 36.1 MG SODIUM

2 cups (medium packed) kale, stems removed
3 cups filtered water
1 cup frozen peaches
2 raw eggs (optional)

*Place all ingredients into a high-powered blender and blend until uniform.
Serve chilled.*

SERVES 2.

Recipe Tidbit:

You can use various greens for this drink. Parsley, collard greens, and spinach are some of my favorites. You can try replacing the peaches with frozen pears. Frozen berries can work well too, but will turn the drink a brownish color. If you are partial to "pretty" food, then I would stick to the peaches or pears. Peaches and pears are low-glycemic-index fruits. This drink is a refreshing option for breakfast. The egg adds protein so it can help to stabilize blood sugar levels.

Green Drink

PER SERVING: 15 CALORIES – 1.2 G PROTEIN – 2.7 G CARBOHYDRATE – 1.3 G FIBER – 0.3 G TOTAL FAT – 0.1 G SATURATED FAT – 0.0 MG CHOLESTEROL – 29.8 MG SODIUM

1 large bunch parsley
3 cups filtered water
2 drops stevia
Lemon juice to taste

Place all ingredients into a high-powered blender and blend until uniform. Serve chilled.

SERVES 3.

Recipe Tidbit:

I suggest trying to make this particular drink 2 times per week and then drinking about a third of it daily. I have been using this same drink for my patients for over a decade with excellent results. Parsley can act as a powerful blood cleanser and supports digestion. It has been rated as one of the plant sources with the highest antioxidant activity. It is high in potassium, calcium, manganese, iron, and magnesium. It is also high in vitamin A, vitamin C, vitamin E, vitamin K, beta-carotene, zeaxanthin, lutein, cryptoxanthins, and folic acid. Fresh herb leaves are also rich in many essential vitamins such as pantothenic acid (vitamin B5), riboflavin (vitamin B2), niacin (vitamin B3), pyridoxine (vitamin B6), and thiamine (vitamin B1).

Protein Fiber Blender Drink

PER SERVING: 327 CALORIES – 9.7 G PROTEIN – 8.3 G CAR-
BOHYDRATE – 6.0 G FIBER – 28.9 G TOTAL FAT – 13.2 G
SATURATED FAT – 0.0 MG CHOLESTEROL – 180.3 MG SODIUM

1 cup unsweetened almond milk (homemade is best)
1 tablespoon flax seeds
2 tablespoons hemp seeds
1 tablespoon coconut oil
½ teaspoon vanilla extract
½ teaspoon cinnamon
Pinch nutmeg

*Place all ingredients into a high-powered blender and blend until uniform.
Drink immediately.*

SERVES 1.

Recipe Tidbit:

This drink is power packed with protein but not very sweet. Get used
to enjoying the nutty flavor of seeds and nuts without needing the
sweetness. This drink can satisfy your appetite for a couple of hours
and should be used as a snack or accompaniment to a meal. If you
want the drink to be heartier so it will stay with you longer, add 1 raw
egg and ½ an avocado. Because of the seed content of this smoothie
it is best if you drink it right away. If it is left to sit, it will thicken
and not be as palatable.

Homemade Almond Milk

PER SERVING: 91.4 CALORIES – 3.4 G PROTEIN – 3.4 G CARBOHYDRATE – 1.9 G FIBER – 7.9 G TOTAL FAT – 0.6 G SATURATED FAT – 0.0 MG CHOLESTEROL – 3.3 MG SODIUM

1 cup organic whole almonds, blanched, skins removed (see below)
1 cup hot water
3 cups room-temperature water

Blend almonds with hot water in a blender until very smooth. Add remaining 3 cups water and process until very smooth. Strain through cheesecloth into a glass container. Refrigerate.

YIELDS 4 1/2 CUPS (9 1/2-CUP SERVINGS).

Kitchen Tip:

Blanch almonds by boiling them in water for 1–2 minutes. Then drain, cool, and pinch off the skins.

Substitutions:

You can try this recipe with various seeds, soybeans, or other nuts. Nuts with skins, such as Brazil nuts and hazelnuts, should be blanched and skins removed. Cashews can be used with no blanching. Some recipes call for soaking the almonds overnight, but making almond milk on the fly is possible when you blanch them. So easy! You can add vanilla extract or a mild sweetener if desired.

Kitchen Tip:

Making your own nut milks saves a lot of money. I don't always make my own, but I love knowing how to do so. I usually have nuts or seeds in my refrigerator that I can use in a pinch to make milk. For certain recipes, such as tapioca pudding, I prefer making the milk myself because I feel that fresh milk makes a much better-tasting product. Same thing with flours: if a recipe calls for flour, I always have grains on hand that I can grind into a fine flour. You can do this easily in a coffee grinder or in a high-powdered blender or food processor.

White Bean Hummus

PER SERVING: 58.1 CALORIES — 3.0 G PROTEIN — 7.2 G CARBOHYDRATE — 2.1 G FIBER — 2.3 G TOTAL FAT — 0.3 G SATURATED FAT — 0.0 MG CHOLESTEROL — 98.4 MG SODIUM

Making this recipe one day ahead of time helps the flavors marry and intensify.

> 3 cups cooked great northern beans, or 2 15-ounce cans, rinsed and drained
> ½ cup roasted red peppers
> ⅓ cup tahini (sesame seed butter)
> ⅓ cup lemon juice
> ⅓ to ½ cup water
> 3 garlic cloves, minced
> ¾ teaspoon salt
> Pinch cayenne pepper

Process all ingredients in a food processor until smooth.

SERVES 20.

Recipe Tidbit:

Hummus is traditionally made with garbanzo beans. I love substituting any of the white beans because they seem to make a smoother hummus. You can omit the roasted red peppers and cayenne for a plain hummus, to which you can add various seasonings and vegetables such as roasted garlic, artichokes, spinach, or pesto. To save money, for the tahini, you can substitute 1 teaspoon sesame oil plus 1 teaspoon finely ground sesame seeds.

Protein Delight Seed Crackers

PER SERVING: 263 CALORIES – 9.9 G PROTEIN – 13.6 G
CARBOHYDRATE – 8.3 G FIBER – 20.4 G TOTAL FAT – 2.6 G SAT-
URATED FAT – 46.5 MG CHOLESTEROL – 173.5 MG SODIUM

¼ cup chia seeds
¼ cup sunflower seeds
¼ cup flax seeds
½ cup sesame seeds
1 cup water
1 organic egg
¼ teaspoon sea salt
¼ teaspoon pepper
¼ teaspoon rosemary
½ teaspoon thyme
2 cloves garlic, minced fine
1 shallot, minced fine

Preheat oven to 350 degrees. Combine all ingredients in a large bowl. Line a 9 x 13–inch baking sheet with parchment paper, making sure the parchment paper overlaps the edges of the pan as the mixture will be liquid and will spread to the edges. Pour entire mixture onto the parchment paper and spread evenly. Bake for 30 minutes. Remove the pan and carefully cut into 1-2-inch crackers. Flip each cracker over and bake for another 20 minutes until crispy on the edges. Remove from heat and spatula the crackers onto a baking cloth to dry. When completely cool, transfer to an airtight container.

SERVES 4.

Recipe Tidbit:

The power of seeds! Seeds are packed with protein and fiber. Additionally, on this diet, you may be missing your familiar carbohydrate snacks such as chips and crackers. These little crackers help satisfy that crunchy carbohydrate craving, and they help to fill you up. Furthermore, protein can help to regulate blood sugars. Try using these crackers to dip in hummus or to eat alongside sliced cucumber or yellow beets. You can try various seeds for these crackers and can experiment with different spices as well.

CHAPTER 15

Beyond 30 Days

Foods to Try

I understand that after 30 days, this diet can get a little monotonous, so I have allowed my patients to start adding in some food items after 30 days. You must watch your weight, how you feel, and your blood sugar levels closely. Here are some food items to experiment with:

- Nuts and seeds
  - » Add raw almonds or almond butter.
- Nut butters can be a great additive for smoothies to add protein
  - » Add cashews, pecans, walnuts, and pistachios.
  - » Be careful when consuming nuts that you don't overconsume, which can bring down your appetite. Decreasing your appetite is good, but make sure you don't start replacing your vegetables with nuts.
- Legumes
  - » Try soaking your own black beans, pinto beans, and other types of beans. Beans are high in carbohydrates; therefore you should watch closely to see how you do while consuming beans.

Additionally, beans should be consumed with large amounts of vegetables or over a salad.

- Fruits
  - » Add plums, peaches, nectarines, apricots, grapefruit, and apples.
  - » Pay attention to your weight, blood sugar, and how you feel. Do not replace your vegetables with fruit. Add fruit as a treat only or as an addition to a smoothie, salad, or entrée.

CHAPTER 16

Troubleshooting the Diet

Medication Changes

This is a rather important area to troubleshoot. As you make these changes, if you are currently on diabetic medications, you'll have to watch your blood sugar and how you feel very closely. If your blood sugar levels are around 100 and you're used to them being significantly higher, you may still feel hypoglycemic. If this happens, then you should seek out your doctor to share with him/her your progress and to inquire about weaning you off your medications. It is important to not wean off your medications too quickly and to continue your medications when you start this program.

Involve your doctor if you feel like you need medication changes along the way. If you are using immediate-release insulin, changes in the unit dosage of your insulin can be easily adjusted by taking into account the carbohydrate content of your meal and how much exercise you are doing. Additionally, if you compare what you are eating now to what you were eating before this program, you can better guesstimate where your insulin units should be. If you are a long-time insulin user, this makes sense, and the alterations that you need to make will come easier to you. If you are currently on insulin but haven't been using it for long and therefore haven't had a lot of time to experiment with changing your units, this may pose a difficult and even dangerous problem if your blood sugar levels drop dramatically due to your improved diet. If you are new to insulin, please consult your physician before starting this program so that you are better equipped with the knowledge of how to modify your insulin dosages.

If you are taking immediate-release insulin combined with an extended-release form, it is easiest to keep the extended-release insulin at a consistent dosage while altering only your immediate-release insulin. Consult your physician to be monitored throughout this program so that changes can be made in your insulin if needed. Someone with type 1 diabetes mellitus can adopt these diet changes and reduce their insulin need and see improvement in their health and well-being. Type 2 diabetics can see great results and may sometimes completely eliminate their need for diabetic medications. The changes accomplished by this diet and program can be lifelong if a healthy diet and lifestyle are adhered to after 60 days. If someone is able to get off all their medications and remain faithful to a healthy diet, exercise, and stress management, most likely this person will continue to live day to day without the need for medication.

If you are not using insulin but using another diabetic medication such as metformin, monitor your sugar levels and how you feel. If your blood sugar levels drop significantly, consider reducing your dosage. Your physician can help you reduce your dosage to a level that's comfortable for both of you. Because side effects are often dose dependent, reducing the dosage of a diabetic medication may make you feel a little better if done appropriately once your blood sugar levels have become more normalized. Consequently, reducing your diabetic medications before your blood sugar levels begin to normalize can have a negative impact on how you feel. Make sure you understand what your blood sugar balance is doing before your reduce your dosage.

Blood Sugar Still Too High

At first you may not notice a change in your blood sugar levels even though you are doing all this hard work. Rest assured there is a lot going on underneath that you cannot begin to understand.

Sometimes the failure to maintain diet and lifestyle measures long enough to feel the benefit is why people don't get better and don't stick to programs. What you may not see is that the blood sugar isn't changing much, but other things may be changing. Your insulin may be changing, your insulin response and insulin receptors may be changing, your fat distribution may be changing, your blood vessel healing may be changing, your lipid levels may be changing, and so on. So stick with the program. I have used this diet and program with many patients who have seen significant benefits.

If after 30 days you are still not seeing a change with your blood sugar levels, you should do a few things. First, consult your doctor and explain the program that you are doing and the slow response that you have had. Second, re-examine everything you have been doing. Are you exercising, are you eating enough and often enough, are you sneaking or cheating, are you under a lot of stress, are you having trouble sleeping? Many of these factors and others can affect your response to the therapy. If after 30 days your blood sugar levels haven't changed but you are following the program to a tee, I am going to have you add some antioxidants to your program to help your body better handle oxidative stress.

Supplements to add after 30 days of non-response of blood sugar levels:

- NAC: 600 mg 2 times daily
- Vitamin E: 400 IU per day
- Zinc: 30 mg twice a day (make sure to take with food)

Remember that supplements are not everything. If you aren't sleeping and exercising, then adding these supplements will not be your magic bullet. The body functions as a whole and it heals as a whole. If everything is not in harmony in the chorus, many problems can arise. Trying to supplement the problems away is not the answer.

Blood Sugar Dipping Too Low

If your blood sugar is dipping too low and you are on medications, visit your physician immediately to discuss eliminating or reducing your medication doses. Also, begin to eat smaller meals more often to ensure a better balance of your blood sugar levels. Making sure to include protein with every meal will help you steady your blood sugar levels.

If your blood sugar is dipping too low and you are not on medications, then you need to eat more often or you need to eat more. Check to make sure that you are eating enough. If you feel like you are not eating enough, you can simply add another serving of vegetables at each meal in addition to some protein. Protein snacks in between meals can also help to keep your blood sugar levels balanced.

Not Eating Enough

Believe it or not, this is a common problem among my patients when I put them on the diet. For whatever reason, they start to skip meals or eat unacceptably small portions, and this can throw the body's balance off significantly. Interestingly, if you aren't eating enough, then the body will choose to store any calories as fat because it believes it is in a state of famine. It is the smart, innate survival mechanism we were all born with. We need to move daily, and we need to eat enough for our bodies to remain in balance and to facilitate weight loss if we desire it.

Sometimes I think the problem is that people lose their desire to eat because they don't get to eat the fatty, fried, sweet foods that they are used to. I receive the following common comment, "I just don't really want to eat anymore," or "I have lost all of my yummy food, so nothing seems good to me anymore." This can pose a large problem and can negatively affect your blood sugar and therefore your ability to lose weight, feel better, and decrease aging. My suggestion is to find a few go-to foods that you really like. Experiment with different foods allowed in the diet until you find some good go-tos. A few examples could include celery with unsweetened sunflower butter or carrots with hummus or romaine dipped in hummus or butter lettuce wraps. Anything to get you excited to eat!

Cravings

Cravings for sweets can sometimes be significant, and sweet foods should only be eaten as a complement to your healthy diet. And for this diet, really the only sweet foods that you are allowed to eat are berries. Interestingly, as you eat this diet longer, you'll find that many of the other foods allowed on this diet become very sweet to you. For example, the reason that I allow sweet potatoes and yams on the diet even though they are not low glycemic index is because they taste sweet and can help to curb the sweet cravings that people have. It is innate that we crave sweet. Our body thrives on sugar. In the days before modern diets, our bodies thrived on the caloric density of sugary foods. This reaction was appropriate many years ago when we didn't come across artificially sweetened foods. Now that our diets have changed immensely, we have not evolved out of our sweet tooth. Our brain craves sugar, and now it is overly abundant in our diet. It would be best to go back to the roots of our ancestors. Eat simple and plain foods, and enjoy the natural tastes of food. As we become more deficient in nutrients, I think our taste buds crave more distinctly flavorful foods. If you can increase your nutrient balance and improve your diet, the simple foods will become tastier to you than they were when you first started this diet.

Here are some helpful tips to help you crave sweets less. When you are first craving something sweet, drink a large glass of water and set a timer for 15 minutes. Don't eat the sweet until the timer goes off. You'll sometimes not even want the sweet by time the timer goes off. Also, make sure you are eating regular meals throughout the day and, if needed, having small protein snacks between meals. Skipping meals can increase your cravings for sweets toward the end of the day.

Additionally, make sure that you are eating enough fat. Fat can help curb sweet cravings. You can use oils as salad dressings, eat avocados, coconut, and good fatty fish like salmon. Consuming protein-rich seeds can also help you increase your healthy fat consumption.

Eating Out

When you eat out, consider ahead of time what you are willing to let yourself eat and what you want to accomplish with the meal. Most of the time, the purpose of eating out is to enjoy a party of people socially, even if it is just your family. There is no time spent preparing food or cleaning up, so use this time to enjoy the people you are with. And use this time as a special treat for your soul. If you feel stressed the entire time you are out, you won't digest the food anyway. Most restaurants offer something that you can "cheat" on that won't break the bank. Avoid fast food restaurants and restaurants that serve a lot of fried food.

Here are a few pointers for eating out:

- Order salads. You can even bring your own dressing if needed. Choose salads made with rich, dark greens like spinach or mixed greens rather than iceberg lettuce.
- Order grilled meats and fish with vegetable sides. Skip the potatoes and the bread. Ask them if they can bring you more vegetables or a salad instead.
- Don't let them bring the fries as your side dish because you may just eat them. Order a side salad or side vegetables instead.
- Want a burrito or wrap but don't want the tortilla? Order the insides served like a salad. Ask them to serve the contents as a bowl instead of a burrito. I haven't been to many places that wouldn't do this for me.
- Ask them to leave out the bun or bread that comes with the entrée. Don't let it arrive and think you won't eat it. Take the temptation away before it is there in front of you.
- Skip the "special sauces" if you can, because most likely they will contain dairy, sugar, and gluten.
- Many restaurants now have gluten-free options, which can be very helpful but will still offer a large carbohydrate content. Save these cheats for after your 60-day program and instead order a lettuce wrap.
- Eat a snack containing protein and fat 30 minutes before you go out to help you control your appetite when ordering food. Good choices include avocado, a handful of seeds, or a small handful of raw nuts.
- If you know you are going to be eating out in the evening,

make sure you stay extremely hydrated during the day. Finish drinking half your weight in ounces of water at least 30 minutes before you go to eat.

- To aid digestion of a meal you are unaccustomed to, supplement with one or two capsules of a digestive enzyme before eating. Drinking two teaspoons of apple cider vinegar or one teaspoon of lemon juice in a little bit of water prior to the meal can also stimulate digestive capability.
- This may be a given, but don't order dessert.
- Drink only small amounts of water while you eat. Don't order any sweet drinks.
- If you are dying to have an alcoholic drink, order clear liquor served on the rocks, or with club soda and a lime. And keep it to only one.
- Don't eat out for convenience; eat out for social or family connection. Eating out for convenience means you didn't plan your meals well enough in advance.

Afterword

The human body is powerful and amazingly complex. I cannot stress enough the importance of continuing on this pathway to keep your body healthy for the longest time possible. Sixty days is just your beginning. Many people can go through many diet changes and see response, but if they don't continue the effort, they will end up right back where they started. Don't make the same mistake. Consider this your new ticket to freedom. Your new trick to becoming healthier and staying healthier! Don't give up and don't fret. Don't be hard on yourself if you make a mistake or fall off the wagon. Get up and get back on it. Eating healthier and making good choices are for life now, so if you make some mistakes (as we all do), it is okay, but you should learn from them and move on. Consider this lifestyle and diet change to be your new you, your new way of life, and your new way to accomplish feeling better day to day.

Evolutionarily, we didn't have to put much effort into long-term survival because daily we were putting effort into short-term survival. Hunting and gathering as a society kept our bones and muscles strong and kept our physical brain stimulated. We didn't have the choice of processed, heated, powdered, sugared foods. We ate very simply and didn't have near the toxin load that we have today. Just our daily effort to survive was like traveling upstream. As a species, we had to work hard to live. Now we have the "convenience" of processed foods and sedentary lifestyles. We are making huge intellectual strides at survival, but we have forgotten the physical component to survival as well as the nutritive component of eating healthy, real foods.

As I said before, I like to tell my patients that when they begin this diet and begin turning their health around for the better, it is like turning around a large ship in the water to travel upstream. It is most difficult to initiate the turn, then takes a lot of effort in the beginning to get the ship going in the right direction. Then it will take continued effort forever to keep the ship traveling upstream but should be easier once you have already turned around. If you give up and stop propelling yourself upstream, the ship will turn itself around and travel right back to where you came from. It is the same thing with health. We must always work at it and always put effort into the way we live our lives and the way we feel.

The doctor of the future will give no medicine but will interest his patients in the care of the human frame, in diet and in the cause and prevention of disease.

— THOMAS EDISON

Endnotes

1. Leandro Fornias Machado de Rezende et al. "Sedentary Behavior and Health Outcomes Among Older Adults: A Systematic Review." BMC Public Health 14 (2014): 333. doi:10.1186/1471-2458-14-333.
2. Mai-Lis Hellénius, Carl Johan Sundberg. "Physical Activity as Medicine: Time to Translate Evidence into Clinical Practice." Br J Sports Med 45 no. 3 (2011): 158. doi:10.1136/bjsm.2011.084244.
3. Hannah Arem et al. "Leisure Time Physical Activity and Mortality: A Detailed Pooled Analysis of the Dose-Response Relationship." JAMA Intern Med 175 no. 6 (2015): 959–67. doi:10.1001/jamainternmed.2015.0533; Klaus Gebel et al. "Effect of Moderate to Vigorous Physical Activity on All-Cause Mortality in Middle-Aged and Older Australians." JAMA Intern Med 175 no. 6 (2015): 970–77. doi:10.1001/jamainternmed.2015.0541.
4. Michael Babyak. "Exercise Treatment for Major Depression: Maintenance of Therapeutic Benefit at 10 Months." Psychosom Med 62 no. 5 (September/October 2000): 633–38.
5. Stephanie Doyle. "Modest Exercise Helps Chronic Pain Patients." Medscape, based on abstract 105 presented at the American Academy of Pain Medicine 24th Annual Meeting, February 2008. http://www.medscape.com/viewarticle/570268.
6. Pratik Pimple et al. "Association between Anger and Mental Stress—Induced Myocardial Ischemia." Am Heart J 169 no. 1 (January 2015): 115–21. http://dx.doi.org/10.1016/j.ahj.2014.07.031.
7. Sohyun Park et al. "Factors Associated with Sugar-Sweetened Beverage Intake among United States High School Students." J Nutr 142 no. 2 (February 2012): 306–12. doi:10.3945/jn.111.148536.
8. Kristin Bernard, Ph.D. et al. "Intervention Effects on Diurnal Cortisol Rhythms of CPS-Referred Infants Persist into Early Childhood: Preschool

Follow-up Results of a Randomized Clinical Trial." JAMA Pediatr. 169 no. 2 (February 2015): 112–119.

9. David S. Black et al. "Mindfulness Meditation and Improvement in Sleep Quality and Daytime Impairment among Older Adults with Sleep Disturbances: A Randomized Clinical Trial." JAMA Intern Med 175 no. 4 (2015): 494–501. doi:10.1001/jamainternmed.2014.8081.

10. Caroline Cassels. "Meditation Improves Endothelial Function in Metabolic Syndrome." Medscape, based on abstract 1639 presented at the American Psychosomatic Society (APS) 69th Annual Scientific Meeting, March 10, 2011. http://www.medscape.com/viewarticle/739296.

11. https://www.framinghamheartstudy.org

12. E.D. Eaker et al. "Marital Status, Marital Strain, and Risk of Coronary Heart Disease or Total Mortality: The Framingham Offspring Study." Psychosom Med 69 no. 6 (July-August 2007): 509–13.

13. Cheryl Ulmer, Dianne Miller Wolman, and Michael M. E. Johns, eds., Resident Duty Hours: Enhancing Sleep, Supervision, and Safety (Washington, DC: National Academies Press, 2008).

14. John T. James "A New, Evidence-Based Estimate of Patient Harms Associated with Hospital Care." Journal of Patient Safety 9 no. 3 (September 2013): 122–28. doi:10.1097/PTS.0b013e3182948a69.

15. Francesco P. Cappuccio et al. "Sleep Duration and All-Cause Mortality: A Systematic Review and Meta-Analysis of Prospective Studies." Sleep 33 no. 5 (May 2010): 585–92.

16. http://www.who.int/nutrition/publications/guidelines/sugars_intake/en/.

17. "Be a Sugar Detective." Yale Health. http://yalehealth.yale.edu/sugardetective.

18. Laura O'Connor et al. "Prospective Associations and Population Impact of Sweet Beverage Intake and Type 2 Diabetes, and Effects of Substitutions with Alternative Beverages." Diabetologia 58 no. 7 (2015): 1474–83. doi:10.1007/s00125-015-3572-1.

19. QuanheYang et al. "Added Sugar Intake and Cardiovascular Diseases Mortality among US Adults." JAMA Intern Med 174 no. 4 (2014): 516–24. doi:10.1001/jamainternmed.2013.13563.

20. Shakira F. Suglia, Sara Solnick, and David Hemenway. "Soft Drinks Consumption Is Associated with Behavior Problems in 5-Year-Olds." The Journal of Pediatrics 163 no. 5 (2013): 1323–28. doi:http://dx.doi.org/10.1016/j.jpeds.2013.06.023.

21. Crina Frincu-Mallos. "ENDO 2009: Use of Artificial Sweeteners Linked to 2-Fold Increase in Diabetes." Medscape, based on abstract P2-478 presented at ENDO 2009: The Annual Meeting of the Endocrine Society, June 11, 2009.

http://www.medscape.com/viewarticle/704432.

22. Jotham Suez et al. "Artificial Sweeteners Induce Glucose Intolerance by Altering the Gut Microbiota." Nature 514 (2014): 181–86. doi:10.1038/nature13793.

23. M. Yanina Pepino, Ph.D. et al. "Sucralose Affects Glycemic and Hormonal Responses to an Oral Glucose Load." Diabetes Care 36 no. 9 (2013): 2530-35.

24. Dan Hu et al. "Fruits and Vegetables Consumption and Risk of Stroke: A Meta-Analysis of Prospective Cohort Studies." Stroke 45 (May 2014): 1613–19. doi:10.1161/STROKEAHA.114.004836.

25. http://www.medscape.com/viewarticle/737342_2.

26. Phienvit Tantibhedhyangkul, Sami A Hashim, and Theodore B Van Itallie. "Effects of Ingestion of Long-Chain and Medium-Chain Triglycerides on Glucose Tolerance in Man." Diabetes 16 no. 11 (November 1967): 796–99. doi:10.2337/diab.16.11.796.

27. Jyrki K. Virtanen et al. "Egg Consumption and Risk of Incident Type 2 Diabetes in Men: The Kuopio Ischaemic Heart Disease Risk Factor Study." Am J Clin Nutr 101 no. 5 (April 2015): 1088–96. doi:10.3945/ajcn.114.104109.

28. Artemis P. Simopoulos. "The Importance of the Omega-6/Omega-3 Fatty Acid Ratio in Cardiovascular Disease and Other Chronic Diseases." Exp Biol Med 233 no. 6 (June 2008): 674–88. doi:10.3181/0711-MR-311.

29. R. Janknegt. "Drug Interactions with Quinolones." J Antimicrob. Chemother 26 (1990): 7-29.

30. NVSR, "Deaths: Final Data for 2013," table 10, http://www.cdc.gov/nchs/data/nvsr/nvsr64/nvsr64_02.pdf, quoted in Centers for Disease Control and Prevention, "Faststats: Leading Causes of Death." http://www.cdc.gov/nchs/fastats/leading-causes-of-death.htm.

31. "The Top 10 Causes of Death." World Health Organization. Last modified May 2014. http://www.who.int/mediacentre/factsheets/fs310/en/index2.html.

32. Karen Davis et al. Mirror, Mirror on the Wall: How the Performance of the U.S. Healthcare System Compares Internationally (New York: The Commonwealth Fund, June 2014). http://www.commonwealthfund.org/~/media/files/publications/fund-report/2014/jun/1755_davis_mirror_mirror_2014.pdf.

33. T. Edwards "Inflammation, Pain, and Chronic Disease: An Integrative Approach to Treatment and Prevention." Altern Ther Health Med 11 no. 6 (2005): 20-7.

34. Shelly L. Gray et al. "Cumulative Use of Strong Anticholinergics and Incident Dementia: A Prospective Cohort Study." JAMA Intern Med 175 no. 3 (March 2015): 401–7. doi:10.1001/jamainternmed.2014.7663.

35. Awal Al Husain and Ian N. Bruce. "Risk Factors for Coronary Heart

Disease in Connective Tissue Diseases." Ther Adv Musculoskel Dis 2 no. 3 (June 2010): 145–53. doi:10.1177/1759720X10365301.

36. Wallace B. Lebowitz. "The Heart in Rheumatoid Arthritis (Rheumatoid Disease): A Clinical and Pathological Study of Sixty-Two Cases." Ann Intern Med 58 no. 1 (January 1963): 102–123. doi:10.7326/0003-4819-58-1-102.

37. http://www.med.navy.mil/sites/NMCP2/PatientServices/SocialWork/Documents/GeneralDiabetesFacts.pdf.

38. American Diabetes Association. "Economic Cost of Diabetes in the U.S. in 2012." Diabetes Care 36 no. 4 (April 2013): 1033–46. doi:10.2337/dc12-2625.

39. http://ghr.nlm.nih.gov/glossary=basepair.

40. A. Settin et al. "Association of ACE and MTHFR Genetic Polymorphisms with Type 2 Diabetes Mellitus: Susceptibility and Complications." J Renin Angiotensin Aldosterone Syst (January 2014). doi:10.1177/1470320313516172.

41. Serbulent Yigit et al. "Association of MTHFR Gene C677T Mutation with Diabetic Peripheral Neuropathy and Diabetic Retinopathy." Mol Vis 19 (2013): 1626–30.

42. Suzanne de la Monte et al. "Alzheimer's Disease Is Type 3 Diabetes–Evidence Reviewed." J Diabetes Sci Technol 2 no. 6 (November 2008): 1101–13. doi:10.1177/193229680800200619.

43. William J. Walsh. Nutrient Power: Heal Your Biochemistry and Health Your Brain. (New York: Skyhorse Publishing, 2012).

44. Amy Hess-Fischl. "What Is Insulin? Important Hormone Allows Your Body to Use Sugar (Glucose)." Last modified March 25, 2015. http://www.endocrineweb.com/conditions/type-1-diabetes/what-insulin.

45. Diana Zuckerman. "The Worst New Drug of 2014." National Center for Health Research. Last modified February 2014. http://center4research.org/nrc-in-the-news/worst-new-drug-of-2014/.

46. Poster based on IDF Diabetes Atlas, 6th ed. http://www.idf.org/sites/default/files/Atlas-poster-2014_EN.pdf.

47. Centers for Disease Control and Prevention. "National Diabetes Fact Sheet: National Estimates and General Information on Diabetes and Prediabetes in the United States," 2011 (Atlanta, GA: US Department of Health and Human Services, Centers for Disease Control and Prevention, 2011). http://www.cdc.gov/diabetes/pubs/pdf/ndfs_2011.pdf.

48. Centers for Disease Control and Prevention. "National Diabetes Fact Sheet: National Estimates and General Information on Diabetes and Prediabetes in the United States," 2011 (Atlanta, GA: US Department of Health and Human Services, Centers for Disease Control and Prevention, 2011). http://www.cdc.gov/diabetes/pubs/pdf/ndfs_2011.pdf.

49. Marie Ng et al. "Global, Regional, and National Prevalence of Overweight

and Obesity in Children and Adults During 1980–2013: A Systematic Analysis for the Global Burden of Disease Study 2013." Lancet 384 no. 9945 (August 2014): 766–81. doi:10.1016/S0140-6736(14)60460-8.

50. Ronghua Yang and Lili A. Barouch. "Leptin Signaling and Obesity: Cardiovascular Consequences." Circulation Research 101 (2007): 545–59. doi:10.1161/CIRCRESAHA.107.156596.

51. Jordan Kawano and Rohit Arora. "The Role of Adiponectin in Obesity, Diabetes, and Cardiovascular Disease." J Cardiometab Syndr 4 no. 1 (Winter 2009): 44–49. doi:10.1111/j.1559-4572.2008.00030.x.

52. Claudio Marcocci et al. "Carefully Monitored Levothyroxine Suppressive Therapy Is Not Associated with Bone Loss in Premenopausal Women." J Clin Endocrinol Metab 78 no. 4 (April 1994): 818–23. doi:10.1210/jc.78.4.818; V. Nuzzo et al. "Bone Mineral Density in Premenopausal Women Receiving Levothyroxine Suppressive Therapy." Gynecol Endocrinol 12 no. 5 (October 1998): 333–37. doi:10.3109/09513599809012835; Kaoru Fujiyama et al. "Suppressive Doses of Thyroxine Do Not Accelerate Age-Related Bone Loss in Late Postmenopausal Women." Thyroid 5 no. 1 (February 1995): 13–17. doi:10.1089/thy.1995.5.13.

53. Giorgio Iervasi et al. "Low-T3 Syndrome: A Strong Prognostic Predictor of Death in Patients with Heart Disease." Circulation 107 no. 5 (February 2003): 708–13. doi:10.1161/01.CIR.0000048124.64204.3F.

54. Jenny E. Gunton et al. "Iodine Deficiency in Ambulatory Participants at a Sydney Teaching Hospital: Is Australia Truly Iodine Replete?" Med J Aust 171 no. 9 (November 1999): 467–70. http://www.ncbi.nlm.nih.gov/pubmed/10615339; Stephen A. Hoption Cann. "Hypothesis: Dietary Iodine Intake in the Etiology of Cardiovascular Disease." J Am Coll Nutr 25 no. 1 (February 2006): 1–11. doi:10.1080/07315724.2006.10719508.

55. Shigenobu Nagataki, Kazuo Shizume, and Kiku Nakao. "Thyroid Function in Chronic Excess Iodide Ingestion: Comparison of Thyroidal Absolute Iodine Uptake and Degradation of Thyroxine in Euthyroid Japanese Subjects." J Clin Endocrinol Metab 27 no. 5 (May 1967): 638–47. doi:http://dx.doi.org/10.1210/jcem-27-5-638.

56. Alfred O. Mueck. "Postmenopausal Hormone Replacement Therapy and Cardiovascular Disease: The Value of Transdermal Estradiol and Micronized Progesterone." Climacteric 15 no. S1 (April 2012): 11–17. doi:10.3109/13697137.2012.669624.

57. Alfred O. Mueck. "Postmenopausal Hormone Replacement Therapy and Cardiovascular Disease: The Value of Transdermal Estradiol and Micronized Progesterone." Climacteric 15 no. S1 (April 2012): 11–17. doi:10.3109/13697137.2012.669624.

58. Paresh Dandona and Matt T. Rosenberg. "A Practical Guide to Male Hypogonadism in the Primary Care Setting." Int J Clin Pract 64 no. 6 (May 2010): 682–96. doi:10.1111/j.1742-1241.2010.02355.x.

59. Kay-Tee Khaw et al. "Endogenous Testosterone and Mortality Due to All Causes, Cardiovascular Disease, and Cancer in Men: European Prospective Investigation into Cancer in Norfolk (EPIC-Norfolk) Prospective Population Study." Circulation 116 no. 23 (December 2007): 2694–701. doi:10.1161/CIRCULATIONAHA.107.719005.

60. T. Wolden-Hansen et al. "Daily Melatonin Administration to Middle-Aged Male Rats Suppresses Body Weight, Intraabdominal Adiposity, and Plasma Leptin and Insulin Independent of Food Intake and Total Body Fat." Endocrinology 141 no. 2 (February 2000): 487–97. doi:http://dx.doi.org/10.1210/endo.141.2.7311.

61. Ciaran J. McMullen. "Melatonin Secretion and the Incidence of Type 2 Diabetes." JAMA 309 no. 14 (April 2013): 1388–96. doi:10.1001/jama.2013.2710.

62. Er-Yuan Liao et al. "Age-Related Bone Mineral Density, Accumulated Bone Loss Rate and Prevalence of Osteoporosis at Multiple Skeletal Sites in Chinese Women." Osteoporosis Int 13 no. 8 (August 2002): 669–76. doi:10.1007/s001980200091.

63. Edward Giovannucci. "25-Hydroxyvitamin D and Risk of Myocardial Infarction in Men: A Prospective Study." Arch Intern Med 168 no. 11 (June 2008): 1174–80. doi:10.1001/archinte.168.11.1174.

64. American Diabetes Association. "Genetics of Diabetes." Last modified May 20, 2014. http://www.diabetes.org/diabetes-basics/genetics-of-diabetes.html#sthash.y76bwrU7.dpuf.

65. Johannes Hebebrand and Anke Hinney. "Environmental and Genetic Risk Factors in Obesity." Child Adolesc Psychiatr Clin N A 18 no. 1 (January 2009): 83–94.

66. AL Culver et al. "Statin Use and Risk of Diabetes Mellitus in Postmenopausal Women in the Women's Health Initiative." Arch Intern Med 172 no 2. (2012): 144-52. doi: 10.1001/archinternmed.2011.625. Epub 2012 Jan 9.

67. http://www.fda.gov/Drugs/DrugSafety/ucm293101.htm#sa.

68. Caroline Cassels. "High-Protein Diet Linked to Lower Brain Mass in Alzheimer's Mouse Model." Medscape. Published online October 21, 2009. http://www.medscape.com/viewarticle/711217.

69. Y. Gu et al. "Nutrient Intake and Plasma β-amyloid." Neurology 78 no. 23 (June 2012): 1832–1840. doi:10.1212/WNL.0b013e318258f7c2. Deborah Gustafson et al. "Dietary Fatty Acids (FA) and Dementia: Observations from the Washington Heights and Inwood Columbia Aging Project." Alzheimer

Dement 7 no. S (2011): S296–S297. doi:10.1016/j.jalz.2011.05.863.

70. P.K. Elias et al. "Serum Cholesterol and Cognitive Performance in the Framingham Heart Study." Psychosom Med 67 no 1. (2005): 24-30.

71. William Knowler et al. "Reduction in the Incidence of Type 2 Diabetes with Lifestyle Intervention or Metformin." N Eng J Med 346 no. 6 (February 2002): 393–403. doi:10.1056/NEJMoa012512.

72. Nancy Babio et al. "Mediterranean Diets and Metabolic Syndrome Status in the PREDIMED Randomized Trial." CMAJ 186 no. 17 (October 2014): 649–57. doi10.1503 /cmaj.140764.

73. Nalini Ranjit et al. "Psychosocial Factors and Inflammation in the Multi-Ethnic Study of Atherosclerosis." Arch Intern Med 167 no. 2 (January 2007): 174–81. doi:10.1001/archinte.167.2.174.

74. Michael Reece et al. "National Survey of Sexual Health and Behavior." Center for Sexual Health Promotion. Copyright 2010. Nationalsexstudy. indiana.edu; Stuart Brody. "The Relative Health Benefits of Different Sexual Activities." The Journal of Sexual Medicine 7 no. 4.1 (2010): 1336–61. doi:10.1111/j.1743-6109.2009.01677.x.

75. National Center on Addiction and Substance Abuse at Columbia University. National Survey of American Attitudes on Substance Abuse XVI: Teens and Parents. (New York: CASA Columbia, 2011.)   http://www.casacolumbia.org/addiction-research/reports/national-survey-american-attitudes-substance-abuse-teens-parents-2011.

76. Salynn Boyles. "Air Pollution Linked to Risk of Diabetes." WebMD Health News. Last modified October 5, 2010. http://www.medscape.com/viewarticle/729946. Zorana J. Andersen et al. "Chronic Obstructive Pulmonary Disease and Long-Term Exposure to Traffic-Related Air Pollution: A Cohort Study." Am Journal Respir Crit Care Med 183 no. 4 (February 2011): 455–61. doi:10.1164/rccm.201006-0937OC. Jaime E. Hart et al. "Exposure to Traffic Pollution and Increased Risk of Rheumatoid Arthritis." Environmental Health Perspectives 117 no. 7 (2009): 1065–69. doi:10.1289/ehp.0800503.

77. Anne C. Steinmann. "Fragranced Consumer Products and Undisclosed Ingredients." Environ Impact Assess Rev 29 no. 1 (January 2009): 32–38. doi:10.1016/j.eiar.2008.05.002.

78. California Air Resources Board (CARB). Report to the California Legislature: Indoor Air Pollution in California (Sacramento, CA: California Environmental Protection Agency, 2005). http://www.arb.ca.gov/research/apr/reports/l3041.pdf.

79. William W. Nazaroff and Charles J. Weschler. "Cleaning Products and Air Fresheners: Exposure to Primary and Secondary Air Pollutants." Atmospheric Environment 38 no. 18 (June 2004): 2841–65. doi:10.1016/j.

atmosenv.2004.02.040.

80. "EWG'S Dirty Dozen Guide to Food Additives." EWG. Last modified November 12, 2014. http://www.ewg.org/research/ewg-s-dirty-dozen-guide-food-additives.

81. "Fish Consumption Advisories." US Environmental Protection Agency. Last modified December 29, 2014. http://www.epa.gov/hg/advisories.htm.

Recommended Websites and Books

Dr. Jessica Black
www.drjessicablack.com
The author's website offers health tips, cooking tips, and weekly menu planners that can be e-mailed directly to you. It also includes a blog dedicated to exploring ideas for following an anti-inflammatory diet and lifestyle. The Freedom Diet supplement is also available here.

A Family Healing Center
www.afamilyhealingcenter.com
The website of Drs. Jason and Jessica Black's naturopathic medical clinic.

American Association of Naturopathic Physicians
www.naturopathic.org
The official site for the national organization of naturopathic physicians. It offers useful information about naturopathy and will help you find doctors in your area.

Azure Standard
www.azurestandard.com
At this website you can order many bulk and natural foods at lower prices than if you were to purchase them in stores. It requires a minimum order, but you can join others in your area to collectively place orders.

Bastyr University
www.bastyr.edu
Naturopathic medical school located in Seattle, Washington.

The Center for Food Safety
www.truefoodnow.org
A nonprofit organization that offers resources on current eating trends and how to embrace healthier dietary habits.

Centers for Disease Control and Prevention
www.cdc.gov
Offers information about diseases, disease prevalence, acute disease outbreaks, vaccinations, and much more.

The Chopra Center
www.chopra.com
A site for learning how to balance body, mind, and spirit.

Coconut Research Center
www.coconutresearchcenter.com
Information on the coconut.

Eating with Purpose
www.eatingwithpurpose.com
Real-life solutions to eating real food.

Elana's Pantry
www.elanaspantry.com
Gluten-free recipes.

Empowered Sustenance
www.empoweredsustenance.com
Great site offering health tips, recipes, and advice. Skip the baked goods.

Environmental Protection Agency
www.epa.gov

Offers current advice relating to foods, environmental concerns, and much more. The mission of this governmental agency is to protect human health and the environment.

Environmental Working Group
www.ewg.org
Wonderful site on environmental toxins, how they are present in our surroundings, and what you can do to limit exposure.

Fly Lady
www.flylady.net
A site for helping women to stop procrastinating and to create better lifestyle habits.

GAPS Diet
www.gapsdiet.com
Information about the GAPS (Gut and Psychology Syndrome) diet. Includes recipes.

Glycemic Index
www.glycemicindex.com
Easy way to look up glycemic index of foods. It can help you choose foods with a lower GI so that you feel more full and can control your appetite better.

Herb Fusion, LLC
www.herb-fusion.com
Offers physician-designed herbal products for energy, sleep, stress, and general health. Dr. Black and her husband have developed these products based on their years of experience treating patients in their clinic.

Keeper of the Home
www.keeperofthehome.org
Great GAPS ideas and recipes.

Know the Cause
www.knowthecause.com

Information on potential causes of health problems. *Know the Cause* is also a television show hosted by Doug Kaufmann.

Livestrong
www.livestrong.org
This website will soon become a favorite. It provides reliable, up-to-date, researched health information on almost anything you have questions about.

Mayo Clinic
www.mayoclinic.com
A site to help you learn more about various conditions and the current allopathic approach to treating them. The site even supplies some information regarding natural treatments.

Mothering Magazine
www.mothering.com
This is a great site that helps people with similar interests connect around topics related to raising children. People share information and even kefir grains and kombucha scobies through this network.

National College of Naturopathic Medicine
www.ncnm.edu
Naturopathic medical school located in Portland, Oregon, and the school from which the author and her husband graduated.

National Library of Medicine
www.nlm.nih.gov
Operated by the federal government, this is the premier library of health information. Use it to access articles, journals, and other health resources for specific information.

North Carolina State University Cooperative Extension: Pickle and Pickle Product Problems
http://fbns.ncsu.edu/extension_program/documents/foodsafety_pickle_problems.pdf
Food safety sheet on fermenting and pickling foods.

Nourishing Days
www.nourishingdays.com
Great recipes and some information on fermenting.

Oregon Association of Naturopathic Physicians
www.oanp.org
Oregon's state organization for naturopathic physicians. This site can help you locate a physician in your area of the state.

Spunky Coconut
www.thespunkycoconut.com
Offering gluten-free, dairy-free, and paleo recipes. Avoid the baked goods.

Thrive Market
www.thrivemarket.com
Online store for natural items. There is a monthly fee to buy discounted products.

Quick Workouts
http://well.blogs.nytimes.com/2013/05/09/the-scientific-7-minute-workout/
https://www.youtube.com/watch?v=Jru5B044HOs (video of the workout above)
https://www.youtube.com/watch?v=PWEdJRRndkQ (10-minute workout video)

HELPFUL BOOKS

Black, Jessica. *The Anti-Inflammation Diet and Recipe Book: Protect Yourself and Your Family from Heart Disease, Arthritis, Diabetes, Allergies—and More.* 2nd ed. Nashville, TN: Turner Publishing, 2015

Black, Jessica, and Dede Cummings. *Living with Crohn's and Colitis: A Comprehensive Naturopathic Guide for Complete Digestive*

Wellness. Long Island City, NY: Hatherleigh Press, 2010.

Black, Jessica. *More Anti-Inflammation Diet Tips and Recipes.* Alameda, CA: Hunter House, 2013.

Brantley, Jeffrey. *Calming Your Anxious Mind: How Mindfulness and Compassion Can Free You from Anxiety, Fear, and Panic,* 2nd ed. Oakland, CA: New Harbinger Publications, 2007. This book offers concrete suggestions on how to begin a meditation practice and break the habitual thinking that can lead to anxieties.

Crowley, Chris, and Henry S. Lodge. *Younger Next Year: Live Strong, Fit, and Sexy—Until You're 80 and Beyond.* New York: Workman Publishing Company, 2007. This is a great book to help motivate you to exercise.

Eden, Donna. *Energy Medicine: Balancing Your Body's Energies for Optimal Health, Joy, and Vitality.* New York: Tarcher, 2008. An excellent book that offers many ideas on daily tapping routines to increase the flow of energy in the body and to help make healing possible.

Fallon, Sally. *Nourishing Traditions: The Cookbook That Challenges Politically Correct Nutrition and the Diet Dictocrats,* rev. and updated 2nd ed. White Plains, MD: NewTrends Publishing, 2003. A great cookbook and an excellent resource for making fermented foods.

Gates, Donna, and Linda Schatz. *The Body Ecology Diet: Recovering Your Health and Rebuilding Your Immunity.* Carlsbad, CA: Hay House, 2011. First published 2006 by B.E.D. Publications. Discusses increasing gastrointestinal resistance and overall health through the use of probiotics.

Gottschall, Elaine Gloria. *Breaking the Vicious Cycle: Intestinal Health through Diet.* Baltimore, MD: Kirkton Press, 1994. Investigates the link between food and intestinal disorders such as Crohn's disease, ulcerative colitis, diverticulitis, celiac disease, cystic fibrosis, and chronic diarrhea.

Kamm, Laura Alden. *Intuitive Wellness: Using Your Body's Inner Wisdom to Heal.* New York: Atria Books/Beyond Words, 2006. A remarkable memoir about Kamm's health journey.

Kinderlehrer, Jane. *Confessions of a Sneaky Organic Cook, or How to Make Your Family Healthy When They're Not Looking!* New York: New American Library, 1972. Although older, this book contains many good ideas. You can probably find an inexpensive used copy online.

Lair, Cynthia. *Feeding the Whole Family: Cooking with Whole Foods,* 3rd ed. Seattle, WA: Sasquatch Books, 2008. This fun book provides many ideas for quick family meals.

Lipton, Bruce H. *The Biology of Belief: Unleashing the Power of Consciousness, Matter and Miracles,* rev. ed. Carlsbad, CA: Hay House, 2008. A great book on how emotions and thoughts can control your destiny.

Remen, Rachel Naomi. *Kitchen Table Wisdom: Stories That Heal,* 10th anv. ed. New York: Riverhead Books, 2006. Explores the spiritual dimension of the healing arts.

Santorelli, Saki. *Heal Thy Self: Lessons on Mindfulness in Medicine.* New York: Three Rivers Press, 2000. A collection of inspirational essays and meditations used in Santorelli's eight-week course on mindful awareness, available to both healing professionals and patients. Santorelli is the director of the Stress Reduction Clinic at the University of Massachusetts Medical Center.

Index

Acanthosis nigricans, 74
Adiponectin, 100
Adrenal glands, 14, 112–113, 170–171
AGEs (advanced glycation end products), 23, 93–95, 130
Aging, 6–7, 10, 15, 16, 23, 93–95, 103, 113, 121, 139–140, 149
ALA (alpha-linolenic acid), 65
Allergies, 49–50, 61–63, 64
Almond Milk, Homemade, 230–231
Alpha-linolenic acid (ALA), 65
Aluminum additives, 182–183
Alzheimer's disease, 16, 20, 54, 58, 81–82, 114, 120, 121, 137–139
American Heart Association, 26, 27, 127
Animal products, 151
    cooking methods for, 93–95
    cured meats, 180
    farming practices, 42–43, 195
    inflammation and, 64–65
    organic meats, 34–35, 153, 194–195
    See also Dairy products; Eggs
Anti-inflammation drugs, 65, 67–68
Anti-inflammatory diet, 8–9, 39, 64–65, 92, 138, 144
Antibiotics, 41, 42, 50, 194, 195
Anticholinergic drugs, 62

Antihistimines, 62
Antioxidants, 45, 79, 80–81, 120
Apolipoprotein A1 (Apo A1), 133
Apolipoprotein B (Apo B), 133
Appetite, loss of, 242
Arachidonic acid, 64–65
Aromatase, 71, 122
Artificial coloring, 182
Artificial flavoring, 181–182
Artificial sweeteners, 27, 28–30
Arugula and Hummus with Warmed Ground Beef, 215–216
Arugula Topped with Avocado and Salsa, Poached Egg over, 205

Beverages, 14, 25, 26–28, 153–156, 204, 227–230. See also Water
BHA (butylated hydroxyanisole), 181
BHT (butylated hydroxytoluene), 181
Blood sugar, elevated, 38, 41, 161
    glycemic index and, 30–31, 138
    high-sugar diet and, 24–28, 91–93
    inflammation and, 91–95
    metabolic syndrome and, 70–72
    stress, related to, 15
    troubleshooting, 239–241
    See also Diabetes; Insulin resistance; Prediabetes

BNP (brain natriuretic peptide), 134
Bone health, 105, 114, 119–120, 121
Brain natriuretic peptide (BNP), 134
Breakfast, importance of, 175
Breakfast recipes, 203, 205–210
Breast cancer, 71, 85, 109, 113, 114, 117, 122, 124
Bromide toxicity, 111
Brooding, 178
Butylated hydroxyanisole (BHA), 181
Butylated hydroxytoluene (BHT), 181

C-reactive protein (CRP), 144
Caffeine, 14
Cancer, 4, 20–21, 54, 56, 71, 85, 109, 113, 117, 120, 122, 124, 127
Canned food, 150, 195, 196
Canola oil, 36
Carbohydrates, 30, 31, 69, 155
Cardiovascular disease, 123–124
    anti-inflammation drugs, 68
    dietary and lifestyle factors, 13–14, 17, 20–21, 27, 31, 33–39, 144
    elevated blood sugar and, 93
    hormones and, 99–100, 104, 105, 106–107, 108, 114–115, 120, 121
    inflammation and, 58, 66, 93
    as leading cause of death, 54, 55–56
    metabolic syndrome and, 71, 98
    MTHFR mutation, 78, 80
    tests for, 124–136
    See also Cholesterol, high
Celebrex, 68
Chewing, 173
Chia Seed Pudding with Blueberries, 210
Children, 57, 62, 117, 200
    healthy development of, 45–47
    lifestyle habits of, 14–19, 167, 174–175

obesity in, 24, 27, 123
    sugar consumption by, 14, 24, 26–28, 46, 131–132
    toxic exposure, 184–185
Chili, Green Chicken, 225–226
Cholesterol, high, 31, 35, 37–38, 58, 71, 132–133, 134–139
Chromium, 191–192
Chronic pain, exercise for, 12
Cigarettes, 179, 185–186
CLA (conjugated linoleic acid), 195
Cleaning products, 179–180
Coconut oil, 35–36
Conjugated linoleic acid (CLA), 195
Cooking methods, 34, 93–95
Cooking tips, 199–200, 212
Cooking with oils, 34, 35–37
Cortisol, 14–15, 106, 135, 161
COX-2 inhibitors, 68
Crackers, Protein Delight Seed, 234–235
Cravings, 187–188, 243
CRP (C-reactive protein), 144
Cup analogy, 6–9
Cyclooxygenase pathways, 65, 68
Cytokines, 60, 121

Dairy products, 34, 64–65, 152
Death, leading causes of, 54–56
Dehydrated foods, 150
Dementia, 10, 62, 121, 133–134. See also Alzheimer's Disease
Depression, 11–12, 16, 55, 62
DHA (docosahexaenoic acid), 65
Diabetes
    Alzheimer's disease and, 81
    as leading cause of death, 54, 56
    medication adjustments for, 87, 155, 239–240
    medications for, 82–89, 144
    overview, 74–75
    statin drugs, linked to, 136
    tests for, 76, 94–95, 128–132

See also Blood sugar, elevated;
  Insulin resistance; Prediabetes;
  specific type of diabetes
Diabetes mellitus type 1, 75–76, 82,
  121–122, 240. *See also* Diabetes
Diabetes mellitus type 2, 38, 70
  artificial sweeteners and, 27,
    28–30
  coconut oil for, 36
  dry cooking methods, 93–95
  family history and, 77, 123
  high-sugar diet and, 23, 24, 27, 46,
    91–93, 131–132
  hormones and, 71, 114, 115, 119,
    120–122
  lifestyle factors, 10–11, 15, 21,
    177–178
  MTHFR defect, 80–81, 85
  overview, 76–77
  prevention/reversal of, 46, 58,
    86–87, 144
  See also Blood sugar, elevated;
    Diabetes; Insulin resistance;
    Prediabetes
Diacetyl, 182
Diet
  imbalances in, 21–39
  importance of, 5
  unhealthy, negative effects of, 5–6,
    137–138, 139–140
  See also Anti-inflammatory diet;
    Freedom Diet
Dieting, 25, 102
Dinner recipes, 204, 219–226
Docosahexaenoic acid (DHA), 65
Drinks. *See* Beverages
Drugs, 5–6, 185–186. *See also*
  Pharmaceutical medications

Eating out, 243–245
EFAs. *See* Essential fatty acids
Eggs, 37–38, 201
  recipes for, 205, 208–209, 227

Eicosanoids, 63–65
Eicosapentaenoic acid (EPA), 65
Electronic media, 17–20, 160
Elimination and challenge diet,
  151–153
Emotional eating, 186
Emotional health, 4, 41
  exercise, benefits of, 11–12
  GI tract, role of, 51–52
  habits to avoid, 178–179
  hormones and, 103, 112, 115, 120
  inflammation and, 55, 62, 63, 169
  media, impact of, 17–20, 160
  self-medicating, 185–186
  stress relief, 16, 19–20, 165–171
  See also Sleep; Stress
Endocrine system, 102–103, 106
Endorphins, 11, 33, 186
Endothelial function, 16
Energy, balance of, 25, 71–72
Energy drinks, 14
Energy, in food, 149–150
Environmental Protection Agency
  (EPA), 184, 185
Environmental toxins, 110, 116
  cup analogy, 6–9
  metabolism of, 5–6
  sources of, 39–43, 179–185, 195
EPA (eicosapentaenoic acid), 65
Epigenetics, 77
Epinephrine, 112
Erucic acid, 36
Erythrocyte sedimentation rate
  (ESR), 125–126
Essential fatty acids (EFAs), 37, 38–
  39, 45, 64, 137–138, 184, 195, 196
Estrogen, 71, 98, 112–113, 114–117,
  120, 122, 135
Exercise, 71–72
  benefits of, 10, 11–12
  lack of, 9–11, 17, 21, 177–178
  recommendations for, 162–165
Exorphin, 33

Family history, as risk factor, 77, 123–125

Family, impact of media on, 17–18

Family meals, 15, 174–175

Family stress, 15–16

Farming practices, 42–43, 195

Farxiga, 85

Fast foods, 22, 34

Fasting glucose, 73, 76, 128–129

Fasting insulin levels, 131–132

Fat, dietary, 21–22, 33–39, 64, 138, 153–156, 201, 243. *See also* Animal products; Essential fatty acids

Fat storage in body, 25, 72, 242

Fatigue, 14, 16, 104, 112, 113, 118, 170–171

Fiber, 31–32, 91, 92, 229

Fibrinogen, 127–128

Fish, 65, 138, 184–185, 196

Flavor ingredients, 181–182

Food additives, 180–183

Food allergies, 6, 50, 151–153

Food and Drug Administration (FDA), 35, 68, 85, 137, 180–181, 184

Food attitude, 200

Food equipment, 198–199

Food preparation, tips for, 198, 199–200, 212

Food, quality of, 41–43, 150

Framingham heart study, 17, 138–139

Freedom Diet, 25, 144
    benefits of, 86–87, 148–151
    elimination and challenge method, 151–153
    foods to avoid, 155–157, 189
    foods to include, 153–155
    foods to try after 30 days, 235–236
    habits to avoid, 177–189
    habits to include, 159–176

    recipes, 203–235
    troubleshooting, 239–245

Fried foods, 34

Fruits, 31–32, 135–136, 138, 151, 153–156, 195–196, 238

GABA (gamma-aminobutyric acid), 41

GALT (gut-associated lymphatic tissue), 51

Gastrointestinal health, 7, 8, 29, 32, 33, 49–52, 92

Genetic risk factors, 6, 7, 62–63, 77–81, 85, 123–125

Genetically engineered food, 42

Gliadin proteins, 32

Glucophage. *See* Metformin

Glucose Freedom, 191–192

Glutathione (GSH), 79, 80–81

Gluten, 32–33, 50

Glycated hemoglobin, 73, 76, 94–95, 129–131

Glycemic index (GI), 30–31, 138

Glycogen, 25, 69, 72

Glycotoxins. *See* AGEs

Gonads. *See* Sex hormones

Grape seed oil, 37

Green Beans with Salmon, Steamed, 219–220

Green Drink, 228

Green Smoothie, 227

Growth hormone, 42, 103

GSH (glutathione), 79, 80–81

Gut-associated lymphatic tissue (GALT), 51

Habits. *See* Lifestyle habits

HbA1c (hemoglobin A1c), 73, 76, 94–95, 129–131

HDL (high-density lipoprotein) cholesterol, 31, 71, 132–133, 135

Healing, paradigms of, 3–4, 143–145

Health care, comparisons of, 57–58

Heart disease. *See* Cardiovascular disease
Heavy metals, 58, 184–185
Hemoglobin A1c (HbA1c), 73, 76, 94–95, 129–131
Herbal supplements, 44
High-fructose corn syrup, 23–24
High-sensitivity C-reactive protein (hsCRP), 126–127
Histamine, 61–63
Homocysteine, 78–79, 80, 85, 133–134
Hormones, 11, 28, 41, 101–122, 139. *See also specific hormone*
HsCRP (high-sensitivity C-reactive protein), 126–127
Hummus, White Bean, 232–233
Hydrogenated oils, 22, 34
Hyperthyroidism, 104, 110, 111–112
Hypoglycemia, 130, 239, 242
Hypothalamus, 99, 102–103
Hypothyroidism, 104–111

Ibuprofen, 67, 68
IGT (impaired glucose tolerance), 73
Immune cells, 60–61
Immune system, 21, 39, 67
    child development and, 46–47
    coconut oil for, 36
    diabetes and, 75, 81
    gastrointestinal health and, 49–50, 51, 92
    inflammatory processes of, 58–65
    vitamin D, role of, 121–122
Impaired glucose tolerance (IGT), 73
Incretin, 28
Infant mortality rates, 57
Inflammation
    anti-inflammation drugs, 65, 67–68
    chronic diseases, linked to, 53–56, 58, 66, 81, 92–93
    cooking methods and, 34, 93–95

cup analogy, 8–9
dietary fat and, 34, 36, 39, 64–65, 93–95
elevated blood sugar and, 91–95
immune response, role in, 58–65
predominant illnesses and, 53–56
risk factors for, 66–67
stress, linked to, 13–14, 169
tests for, 125–128, 144
vitamin D, role of, 121–122
See also Anti-inflammatory diet
Insulin, for diabetes treatment, 82–83, 155, 239–240
Insulin, function of, 69
Insulin levels, tests for, 76, 128–132
Insulin resistance, 11, 24, 46
    artificial sweeteners and, 28–30
    coconut oil for, 36
    estrogen dominance and, 71
    mechanisms of, 41, 69–70, 102–103
    medications for, 84–85
    melatonin and, 120–121
    metabolic syndrome and, 70–72
    obesity and, 72, 98, 100
    stress, related to, 15
    See also Blood sugar, elevated; Prediabetes
Inulin, 191
Iodine, 109–111, 112

Juice, 26–28, 91

Kale Served with Seasoned Ground Turkey, Steamed, 206–207
Kitchen equipment, 198–199
Kitchen, preparation in, 193–201

Lamb Patty, Parsley, 218
Lauric acid, 36
LDL (low-density lipoprotein) cholesterol, 31, 35, 71, 132–133, 135

Lecithin, 37–38
Legumes, 153–156, 223–224, 232–233, 235–236
Leptin, 99–100
Leukocytes, 60–61
Leukotrienes, 64–65
Lifestyle habits, 139–140
  changing, 86–87, 159–160, 247–248
  mealtimes, 173–176
  negative thinking, 178
  sedentary behavior, 9–11, 17, 21, 177–178
  self-medicating, 185–186
  TV viewing, 21, 167, 177–178
  unhealthy people and, 178–179
  See also Emotional health; Exercise; Sleep
Linoleic acid, 64, 65
Lipid profiles, 31, 71, 132–133
Lipoprotein A (Lp(a)), 133
Lipoprotein-associated phospholipase A2 (Lp-PLA2), 128
Lipoxygenase, 65, 68
Liquid measures, 201
Low-fat diets, 33
Lunch recipes, 203, 211–219
Lymphatic system, 60–61
Lymphocytes, 61

Maillard reaction, 94, 95
Mast cells, 61
MCTs (medium-chain triglycerides), 36
Mealtime habits, 173–176
Measurement conversions, 201
Meats. See Animal products
Media, 17–20, 160
Medications. See Pharmaceutical medications
Medicine, paradigms of, 3–4, 143–145
Meditation, 16, 19–20, 165–166

Mediterranean diet, 37, 144
Medium-chain triglycerides (MCTs), 36
Melatonin, 120–121, 160
Menopause, 113, 118, 139
Mental health. See Emotional health
Mercury exposure, 184–185
Metabolic syndrome, 28, 58, 70–72, 97–98, 120, 144
Metabolism, 5–6, 69
Metformin, 83–85, 88, 144, 240
Microflora, 29, 50
Monolaurin, 36
Monounsaturated fats, 34, 35, 37
MTHFR (methylenetetrahydrofolate reductase) defect, 62–63, 77–81, 85
Myeloperoxidase (MPO), 128

Naproxen, 67, 68
National Institute of Nutrition, 135–136
National Institutes of Health, 21, 81, 120
National Research Center for Women & Families, 85
"Natural flavoring," 181–182
Naturopathic physicians, 143–149
Negative thinking, 178
Nervous system, 12–13, 99, 102
Nitrites/nitrates, 180
NSAIDs (nonsteroidal anti-inflammatory drugs), 67, 68
Nut butters, 237
Nut milks, 230–231
Nutritional supplements, 39, 43–45, 161, 170–171, 191–192, 241
Nuts, 65, 153–156, 213–214, 230–231, 235

Obesity, 97–100
  artificial sweeteners and, 28
  childhood, 24, 27, 123
  fat-storage pathway, 25, 72

gluten and, 32
health risks and prevalence of, 20, 21, 97
hormones and, 98–100, 116–117, 120
lifestyle factors for, 11, 14, 20–21
metabolic syndrome and, 70–72, 97–98
overeating, 186–188
prediabetes, 74
sugar, overconsumption of, 24, 26, 27, 72
See also Weight loss
OGTT (oral glucose tolerance test), 73, 76
Oils, 22, 34, 35–37, 64, 153–154, 156
Olive oil, 34, 35, 36, 37
Omega-3 fatty acids, 37, 38–39, 64, 137–138, 195, 196
Omega-6 fatty acids, 37, 38, 39, 64, 195
Omega-9 fatty acids, 36, 38
Oral glucose tolerance test (OGTT), 73, 76
Oral tolerance, 49
Organic foods, 34–35, 43, 110, 194–196
Osteoporosis. See Bone health
Ovarian cancer, 117
Overeating, 186–188
Oxidative stress, 54, 55, 93, 112, 130, 139–140
Oxytocin, 103, 171

Paleo diet, 35
Palm oil, 37
Pancreatic islet cells, 70, 75
Parasympathetic system, 12–13
Partially hydrogenated oil or fat, 34
Pharmaceutical medications, 8, 106
    anti-inflammatory, 65, 67–68
    antibiotics, 41, 42, 50, 194, 195
    for depression, 11–12

for diabetes, 82–89, 144, 237–238
for histamine reaction, 62
for lowering cholesterol, 136–137, 138–139
metabolism of, 5–6
symptoms, suppression of, 3–4, 46–47
for thyroid, 108–109
Phosphate food additives, 182
Phospholipase A2 (PLA2), 65
Physical trainers, 164–165
Pineal gland, 120–121
Pituitary, 102, 103–104, 105, 107
Polycystic ovarian syndrome, 71, 84–85
Positive affirmations, 168–169
Positive thinking, 4, 166–167, 170
Potassium bromate, 180
Prediabetes, 72–74, 76
Probiotics, 32, 33, 45, 50, 92
Processed foods, 22–24, 31, 32–33, 150, 180, 196
Progesterone, 98, 112–113, 114, 115–118, 135
Propyl gallate, 181
Propyl paraben, 180–181
Prostaglandins, 64–65, 67
Prostate cancer, 113, 117, 120
Protein, 137–138, 153–156
Protein Fiber Blender Drink, 229
Psyllium husk powder, 191

Quinoa Tabouli, 217
Quinolones, 41

Raw foods, 199
Real Salt, 196
Recipes, 203–235
Restaurants, eating in, 243–245
Rheumatoid arthritis, 58, 66, 127, 179

Salmon, Steamed Green Beans with,

219–220
Salt, 109, 196
Saturated fats, 34–38, 138
Secosteroids, 122
Sedentary behavior, 9–11, 17, 21, 177–178
Seeds, 64, 65, 153–156, 213–214, 234–235, 237
Selenium, 111
Self-esteem, 168–169
Self-medicating, 185–186
Serotonin, 51, 79
Sesame oil, 36, 64
"Set point," body weight, 99, 102
Sex hormones, 71, 98, 112–120, 122, 135, 137, 139, 171
Shopping list, 197
Skin tags, 74
Sleep, 13, 14, 16, 18, 20–21, 103, 120–121, 160–162
Smoothie, Green, 227
Snacks, 175–176, 204, 234–235
Social media, 18–19
Soda, 25, 27–28
Spinach Salad with Chicken, Yam, and Goat Cheese, Wilted, 211–212
Statin drugs, 136–137, 138–139
Stevia, 210
Strawberry Green Salad with Pumpkin Seeds, 213–214
Stress, 136, 139–140
    autonomic nervous system and, 12–13
    cholesterol and, 135
    cup analogy, 6–9
    health effects of, 13–16, 169
    hormones and, 14, 15, 112, 113, 117–118
    media, effect of, 17–20
    relief from, 16, 19–20, 165–171
    See also Emotional health
Stress hormone. See Cortisol
Subclinical inflammation, 144

Sugar, dietary, 35, 138
    artificial sweeteners, 27, 28–30
    in beverages, 14, 25, 26–28
    child consumption of, 14, 24, 26–28, 46, 131–132
    cravings for, 187–188, 243
    Freedom Diet and, 25, 156–157
    high-fructose corn syrup, 23–24
    obesity and, 24, 26, 27, 72
    overconsumption of, 24–28, 91–93
    recommended levels of, 25–26
    self-medicating with, 185–186
Supplements. See Nutritional supplements
Sweeteners, artificial, 27, 28–30
Sympathetic system, 12–13
Symptoms, suppression of, 3–4, 46–47

Taco Salad, 221–222
Teenagers, 14, 15, 26, 117, 131–132, 174–175
Television watching, 21, 167, 177–178
Telomeres, 10
Temperatures, cooking, 201
"Terrain," 5, 45–46
Testosterone, 71, 98, 112–113, 118–120, 122, 135, 137, 139, 171
Tests
    for cardiovascular disease, 124–136
    for diabetes, 76, 94–95, 128–132
    for inflammation, 125–128, 144
    for iodine deficiency, 110–111
    for MTHFR defect, 80
    for prediabetes, 73, 76
    for thyroid function, 107–108, 112
Theobromide, 181
Thimerosal, 185
Thyroid function, 104–112
Thyroid-stimulating hormone (TSH), 105, 107–108

Toxins. *See* Environmental toxins
Trans fats, 21–22, 34, 35
Triglycerides, 36, 71, 132, 133,
  134–135
TSH (thyroid-stimulating hormone),
  105, 107–108
Tuna, 185

United States, health care in, 57–58
United States, leading causes of
  death in, 54–55, 56
US Centers for Disease Control and
  Prevention (CDC), 54, 74, 127

Vegetables, 31–32, 35, 135–136, 138,
  153–156, 195–196
Vegetables with Green Lentils,
  Rosemary Roasted, 223–224
Vioxx, 68
Vitamin C, 191–192
Vitamin D, 121–122
Volatile organic compounds (VOCs),
  179–180

Water, 151, 171–172, 173–174, 187,
  194
Weight loss, 31, 36, 86, 98–100,
  148–149, 160, 172, 173
White blood cells, 60–61
White space, 19–20
Whole foods, 151
Women's Health Initiative Trial, 136
World Health Organization
  (WHO), 25–26, 56